Be Your Own Makeup Artist

UNLEASH YOUR INNER BEAUTY.

Natalie Setareh

ISBN: 978-0-5785108-5-9 (ebook)
         978-1-7332718-2-0 (hardcover)
         978-1-7332718-0-6 (paperback)

Front Cover Image and Book Design by Kristin Stokes, Moniker Marketing.
Edited by Kari Perlewitz, Kari Perlewitz Copywriting.

Published by Kindle Direct Publishing, Amazon.

June 2019.

TABLE OF CONTENTS

Be Your Own Makeup Artist

UNLEASH YOUR INNER BEAUTY.

———————————

Natalie Setareh

Hello!

The fact that you're reading these words right now means that you have gone out of your way to find my book and open it up. For that, I thank you so, so, so much. It's people like you who make it possible for me to even have a platform at all to channel all of my makeup and beauty thoughts into. If I didn't have that, I'd just be sharing all this stuff with my husband, and he's already heard enough to write his own book at this point!

I wanted to start by introducing myself a little bit. I'm not a celebrity studded, fashion runway kind of makeup artist. I fell into serving my local community in bridal, lifestyle, corporate, and casual fashion makeup in Monterey, then Augusta, GA, and now Wiesbaden, Germany.

But that's a very brief and incomplete story of how I got to where I am today.

Most people don't know that before my business came into existence, I was a commissioned officer in the United States Air Force. As a matter of fact, I decided to continue my military service part-time in the Air Force Reserves after I separated from Active Duty. Ultimately, I separated from Active Duty service for a number of reasons, but the most important reason was to raise my kids and focus on my family.

Another thing most people don't know? I hold a Masters degree in International Studies! In fact, I started a trade consulting business before I ultimately found my true passion and place in this world as a makeup artist and beauty coach (thank you to all of my dear friends who nudged me down this now very obvious path).

My little makeup business grew quite fast, and after a few years, I realized that my makeup sessions were turning into education sessions. More and more, people wanted private lessons so they could learn more about makeup and it became clear to me that a lot of my clients had the same questions.

Thus, the idea for this book. It's been years in the making. Rather than making money through sponsored content, I have put my head down and worked on building a brand that was trustworthy and unbiased. You'll find that same commitment in these pages you're about to read. Sure, I could have made a ton of money pitching some product I tried once. But I think the world has enough of that.

A final note: this book is written intentionally with gender neutral language because I believe makeup is for everyone. I also believe makeup is multi-generational. This book is meant to make you feel comfortable, so I don't get into the nitty gritty details because I know that's when that "I can't do this" self-doubt creeps in. My goal is to help you feel empowered and confident.

Please join my community on Facebook! As a reader of this book, you are officially invited to join our group called BeYourOwnMUA. I'll be using that space to provide supplemental education, tips, and advice on a regular basis. You can also find me on social media — I'm @nataliesetareh everywhere — and my website is NatalieSetareh.com.

Again, thank you for your support. Now let's dive in!

WELCOME.

THIS GUIDE IS FOR YOU IF YOU HAVE EVER ASKED...

- Do I need to buy all the makeup that I see everyone else using?

- Do I have time to try to learn new makeup techniques?

- Am I too young or too old to change up my makeup routine?

- Why is shopping for makeup so overwhelming and confusing?

- Is makeup even right for me?

I'M NATALIE
AND I BELIEVE...

- Makeup does so much more than just add a bit of color to your face.

- Wanting to feel beautiful isn't selfish, it's human nature!

- With practice and knowledge, we can all become confident in our makeup game!

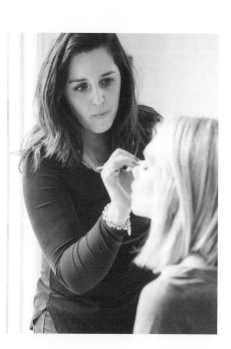

LET'S GET THIS PARTY STARTED!

NO MATTER WHERE YOU ARE IN YOUR MAKEUP JOURNEY, HERE'S WHAT YOU CAN EXPECT FROM THIS BOOK.

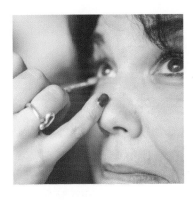

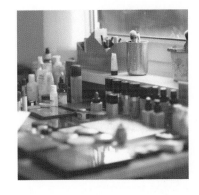

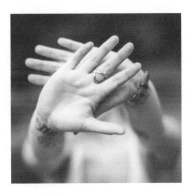

You'll learn the "why" and "how-to" behind YOUR perfect makeup look... not how to imitate someone else's perfect look. Become your own makeup artist!

You'll explore which products and tools are right for you and your specific skin tone and type, and you'll get expert tips (and tricks) for easy and beautiful application.

This book is free of sponsorships and affiliate links. You can find the perfect makeup for any skin type, skin tone, and budget -- all you have to do is know your options.

ARE YOU READY TO BECOME YOUR OWN MAKEUP ARTIST?

DID YOU KNOW...

THESE ARE SOME OF MY FAVORITE FUN FACTS ABOUT MAKEUP.

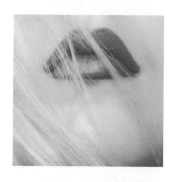

LIPSTICK = WITCHCRAFT

In 1770, British parliament banned lipstick, saying it had the power to seduce men into marriage, which was considered to be witchcraft! [1]

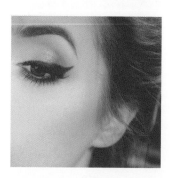

WING LIKE AN EGYPTIAN

The art of painting our faces dates back to 1000 BC in Ancient Egypt. Wearing makeup is practically in our DNA! [2]

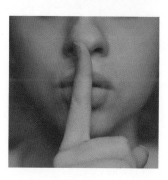

DON'T BELIEVE THE LIES

Not all makeup is bad for your skin! Makeup technology has become so much more sophisticated and now, makeup has some amazing skincare benefits. Wearing makeup can be better than not wearing makeup!

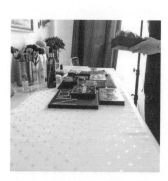

DOUBLE DUTY

You don't need a million products. The right color lipstick can double as blush or eye shadow, matte eye shadows can become brow color, and mixing products you already have can give you tons of new options!

[1] Schaffer, S. (2006, May 19). Reading Our Lips: The History of Lipstick Regulation in Western Seats of Power. Retrieved from dash.harvard.edu/bitstream/handle/1/10018966/Schaffer06.pdf

[2] Eldridge, L. (n.d.). IWonder - The story of make-up. Retrieved from https://www.bbc.com/timelines/z2wk39q

HOW TO USE THIS BOOK

TIP!

You will see this symbol scattered throughout the book. It marks "pro tips" I am sharing to help you improve your makeup selection or application processes.

RESOURCES!

If you see this symbol, I am sharing some of my favorite third-party resources with you. These resources are not sponsored and have been useful in helping me grow my makeup knowledge.

DOUBLE DUTY!

As I mentioned before, many of the products in your makeup kit can pull double duty. I will call those products out throughout the pages that follow by marking them with this symbol.

APPLICATION GUIDE

Different tools work best for different products. I use the symbols below to show my favorite application tools for the products discussed throughout this book. Please note the icons are not indicative of the exact tool.

FINGERTIP APPLICATION

BEAUTY SPONGE

SYNTHETIC BRUSH

NATURAL HAIR BRUSH

THE BUSINESS OF MAKEUP.

There are many makeup brands in the market today, but only a few distributors and manufacturers that actually produce makeup. Knowing the "business" of makeup can help you be a smart consumer and get the most bang for your buck!

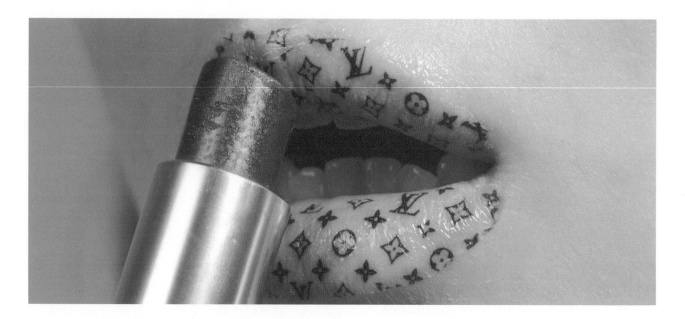

THE (SOMEWHAT UGLY) TRUTH ABOUT BRANDS

Did you know that most makeup brands are part of a larger brand umbrella or conglomerate? This makes shopping for makeup confusing, even for professionals!

If you are someone who tries to shop local and also tries to avoid big box retailers, you're probably aware that multinational corporations like Nestle own many smaller brands (2,000+). Sometimes, the ethics of these large companies are unclear or "shady." The same is true for brands within the beauty industry.

For example, brands like Urban Decay and Ralph Lauren fall under L'Oreal's umbrella... but Nestle owns 30% of L'Oreal. Learning these relationships makes the market feel incredibly small, especially when you start to make these connections. ***Bottom Line: Be a smart consumer!***

USE BRAND KNOWLEDGE TO YOUR ADVANTAGE

Next time you go makeup shopping, keep the list on the following page in mind. For instance, if the foundation you want falls within a larger brand family, you might be able to swap it for another less expensive brand in the same family.

L'OREAL OWNS

Lancôme
Giorgio Armani
Yves Saint Laurent Beauté
Biotherm
Kiehl's
Ralph Lauren
Shu Uemura
Cacharel
Helena Rubinstein
Clarisonic
Diesel
Viktor&Rolf
Yue Sai
Maison Margiela
Urban Decay
Guy Laroche
Paloma Picasso
L'Oréal Paris
IT Cosmetics
Garnier
Maybelline New York
NYX Professional Make Up
African Beauty Brands
Essie
L'Oréal Professionnel
Kérastase
Redken
Matrix
Pureology
Shu Uemura Art of Hair
Mizani
Decléor
CARITA
Vichy
La Roche-Posay
SkinCeuticals
Roger&Galle
CeraVe

ESTEE LAUDER OWNS

Aerin
Aramis
Aveda
Becca
Bobbi Brown
Bumble And Bumble
Clinique
Darphin
Donna Karan New York
Editions De Parfums
Frédéric Malle
Ermenegildo Zegna
Estée Lauder
Glamglow
Jo Malone London
KILLIAN
Kiton
La Mer
Lab Series
Le Labo
M·A·C
Michael Kors
Origins
Rodin Olio Lusso
Smashbox
Tom Ford
Tommy Hilfiger
Too Faced
Tory Burch

LOUIS VUITTON OWNS

Acqua di Parma
Guerlain
Christian Dior
Givenchy
Benefit
Fenty Beauty
Make Up For Ever
Marc Jacobs
Sephora (& many Sephora collabs)
Fresh
Kat Von D

SHISEIDO OWNS

Laura Mercier
NARS
Bare Minerals
Clé de Peau
Majolica Majorca
Serge Lutens
Dolce & Gabbana

COTY OWNS

Rimmel London
New York Color
Burberry
Covergirl
Max Factor
Bourjois
Philosophy
Marc Jacobs (fragrance)
Chloe (fragrance)
Sally Hansen
OPI
Calvin Klein (fragrance)
ghd hair

Key tip! Do your research!

Lots of small brands eventually get bought out by larger brands. It seems to change daily!

This list is current as of 28 May 2019

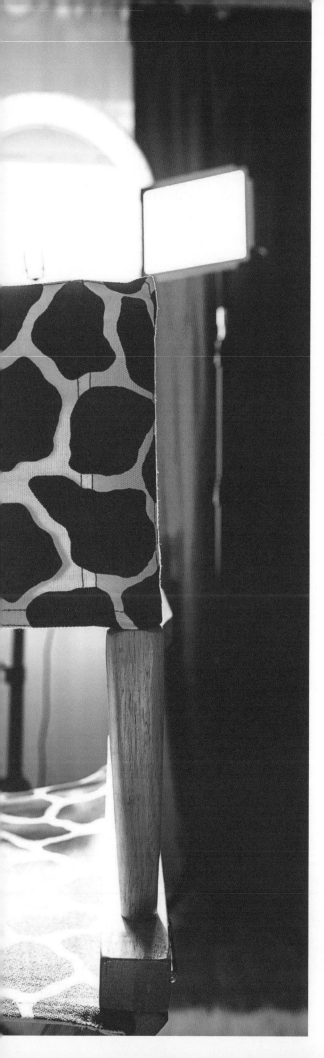

IF IT SEEMS TOO GOOD TO BE TRUE...

IT PROBABLY IS!

BUYER BEWARE!

The counterfeit makeup industry is huge. **Huge!**

- Purchase from official vendors or licensed retailers.
- If the "discount" or price seems too good to be true, walk away (and report them!)
- Craigslist, Ebay, and Amazon are rampant with "gently owned" high-end products and brushes.

If someone posts something like, "I'm selling my mom's old MAC brushes that she never used..." There is a good chance they are FAKE! Con artists sell them for just enough money to make you think they might be real.

WHAT ABOUT DUPES?

Dupes, short for duplicates, **are not counterfeits**. They are products that generally cost less and perform as well as (or similar to) their higher end brand-name counterparts. This is where knowing your brand families can be extremely valuable! Please keep in mind that high end brands may copy smaller, lesser known brands with cult followings, which isn't cool. Again, always do your research if ethics is important to you!

PACKAGING

When you purchase makeup, more times than not, all you're paying for is marketing and packaging. The product's packaging can cost up to THREE TIMES more than the product itself. Consistent skin care, proper makeup application and the right tools (hands and fingers included) are 90%; the actual makeup products are the other 10%. Knowing your brand families may help you to make an educated purchase.

You can really stay in your makeup budget if you learn which products perform similarly at the price point that is right for you!

PRIVATE LABELING

Back in the day, starting your own cosmetics line was something only wealthy people or people with lots of capital could dream of doing. Now, private labeling allows anyone with a few hundred dollars the opportunity to start their own label, but prices increase as customization increases.

HOW IT WORKS

In a nutshell, all you have to do is submit ingredient lists, color formulas, and packaging requests to a private label makeup company, and they will make a batch for a nominal fee. Of course, it's your job to market and sell the products... which is not an easy job!

INFLUENCER & SOCIAL MEDIA MARKETING

When you watch your favorite YouTuber or celebrity test out products on their channels or feeds, know that many of them are either receiving these products for free or are being paid to use them!

Makeup companies (both large and small) learned they don't need to budget for commercial photographers, makeup artists, and models anymore. They can simply send their products to people hoping to receive more "exposure" or "likes" or "subscribers" and save money on marketing. If they do want to splurge, they can pay bigger influencers.

HOW IT HURTS THE MARKET

This practice has resulted in an influx of more photographers, makeup artists, and models working for free, which is undercutting these industries immeasurably! When enough influencers use the same product in ten or twenty different pieces of content, there's enough "social proof" to justify the product's legitimacy. This is a strategic marketing to get consumers to buy. **Period.**

SO WHO CAN YOU TRUST?

It's hard to say! Only you can determine whether someone is authentic or not! Personally, if you have to question whether or not an influencer is being authentic or not when they rave about something, you can probably no longer trust their opinion.

While it's great when someone is upfront about affiliate links, the truth is, it's hard for most people to say something negative about free products. If someone has received something for free, you might want to take their recommendation with a grain of salt. Also, be skeptical about influencers with suspiciously high follower counts. Becoming a "Very Important Person" overnight by buying likes, followers, subscribers, and comments is so incredibly easy and inexpensive. ***Do your research and decide for yourself if their opinion is worth trusting!***

"Beauty
begins the
moment
you decide to
be yourself."

COCO CHANEL

SKINCARE

SKINCARE

THE TRUE FOUNDATION OF IT ALL

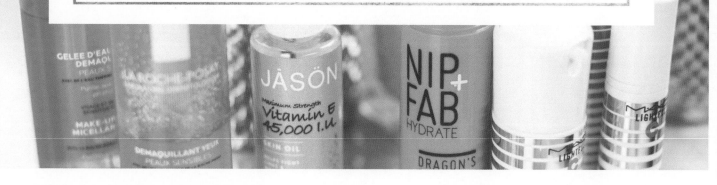

Let me preface this chapter with the disclaimer that I am not an esthetician or a skin care expert. I offer general advice based on my experience working with different skin types throughout the years but if you have specific questions/concerns, it's best to consult with an esthetician or a dermatologist.

There are certain things makeup and a makeup artist can and cannot do. While makeup can do an amazing job of evening out skin tone and reducing the appearance of pores, conventional makeup — we're not talking about special effects makeup here — cannot change the texture of your skin. It cannot make wrinkles disappear, make pores smaller, or make scars invisible.

A proper skincare routine is the #1 area you can focus on to make your makeup look amazing all day, everyday. This the true foundation of any makeup application.

Regardless of what makeup you use, it won't look great on neglected skin. Healthy, glowing skin never goes out of style and good skincare will keep you looking young much longer than no skincare regimen at all.

If your skin has seen better days and you feel like you have to wear makeup to even go outside in public, fortunately for you there are some amazing makeup products that are packed with amazing skincare benefits. You'll learn more about how to seek these products out in the following pages.

YOU'RE NEVER TOO YOUNG OR TOO OLD
TO START TAKING CARE OF YOUR SKIN!

In the next few pages, I'll walk you through the different steps for each skin type, as well as other factors that can impact the health of your skin.

FACTORS AFFECTING SKIN HEALTH

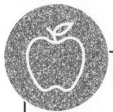

FOOD & H2O

What you eat has an impact on your skin. Try to eat more whole foods and fewer processed foods. Don't forget water, either! You should be drinking at least 48 oz. of water each day for your health and to keep your skin happy!

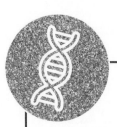

GENETICS

Your DNA is unfortunately one of those factors you can't control. Genetics plays a big role when it comes to your skin type, some skin conditions, and aging in general.

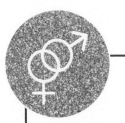

HORMONES

Again, there's not much you can do about hormones, but they can have an effect on your skin's appearance. If you have specific concerns, you can speak to your dermatologist or an esthetician.

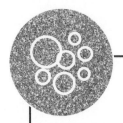

EXFOLIATION

Look at your parents' and grandparents' skin. How did they age? What were the features that aged fastest? Depending on your skin type, you should be using a mild exfoliant to slush away the dead skin cells on your face. This allows for cell rejuvenation and helps in anti-aging.

TIP

Don't forget to take care of your hands and décolletage. These are two areas that are often neglected and show off age too.

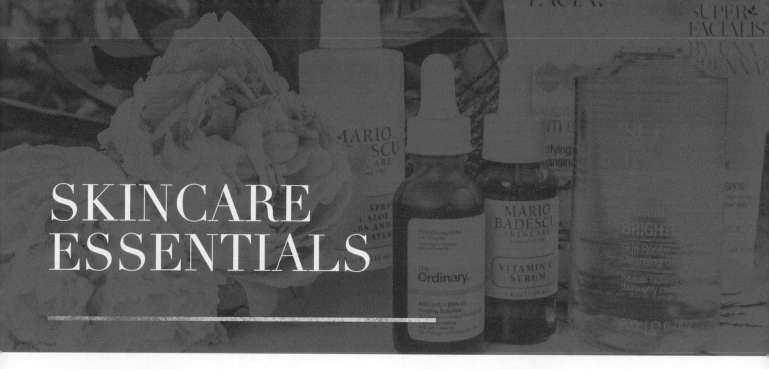

SKINCARE ESSENTIALS

CLEANSING

No matter your skin type, you have to wash your face! You should be washing your face in the morning and in the evening. One of the worst things you can do is go to bed with your makeup on! Not only does this clog your pores but it also **makes your pillowcase dirty** which can lead to acne if you don't wash it regularly. Be sure to choose a cleanser that is formulated for your skin type and you're good to go!

SPF

You should **apply SPF every single day** (chemical or physical), even in wintertime. Some makeup has SPF built-in, and some moisturizers do as well. Otherwise, you can add an SPF to your daily routine for protection from harmful UV rays. Don't worry, most formulas that are on the shelves these days are light, won't clog pores, and don't leave white residue behind. Also know that SPF 30-50 should be sufficient. Anything with SPF higher than 50 has not been scientifically proven to work better than those with SPF between 30 and 50.

MOISTURIZER

Your skin needs moisture to stay youthful. As we get older, we lose elasticity in our skin. Making sure we have enough water in our diet is surely the cheapest and easiest way to take care of our skin, skin — well, that and SPF.

Keeping your skin moisturized, especially at night when it is "at rest" is pure gold in anti-aging. You can buy a decent face moisturizer without spending a ton of money. Look for a formula that addresses your specific skin concerns, and you may also want to add in an **eye cream** for under eye hydration, especially for aging skin. Don't be fooled, though! Eye creams don't reduce dark circles (it's your **genetics** that determine if you have dark circles or not), but they will help keep your under eyes moisturized and thus, your makeup will look better because of it.

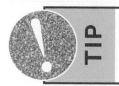

TIP

Your skin type can change as you get older! Pregnancy, stress, hormones, geographic location, water type, and water consumption all play a role. If your makeup has been wearing differently lately, your skin type may be changing.

DETERMINE YOUR SKIN TYPE

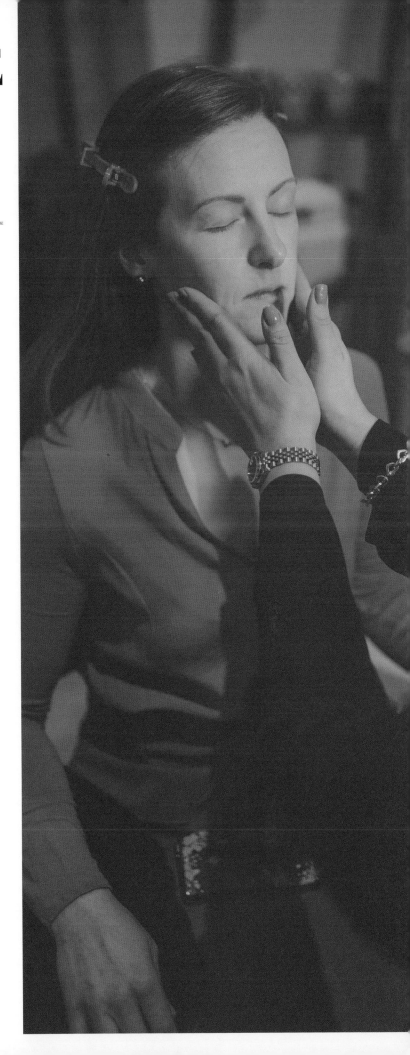

Skin care is extremely important to me, and that is why I want to thank Liz Gardner from Surface by Liz, a professional esthetician and friend for contributing so much helpful information to this chapter.

Knowing your skin type is a vital first step to creating a flattering look. Addressing skin concerns and utilizing a custom skin care routine will ensure that you have the perfect canvas to apply your favorite makeup looks.

If you aren't sure what you skin type is, I have created an interactive guide in this section that pinpoints key features of various skin types.

Work through these pages first before moving into the makeup application section so you know what products will be best for **YOU**!

USING THE SKIN TYPE GUIDE

The skin type guide in the following section will indicate what types of products to look out for!

Feel free to check off characteristics and make notes about your skin type as you work through these pages! The goal for this resource is to help you understand how your skin type can impact how different products perform on your skin.

DO I HAVE

OILY SKIN?

The characteristics listed below are **most commonly associated with oily skin**. Check off the items on the list that accurately describe your skin to see if this is your skin type. If you check most of the boxes, this is most likely your skin type, so **look for products recommended for oily skin** throughout the rest of this book.

YOU MAY HAVE OILY SKIN IF:

○ You see or feel a **layer of oil** on your face in the morning

○ Your face gets **shiny** throughout the day

○ Your face always feels like it needs to be cleansed

○ Your makeup tends to slide off throughout the day

○ You need powder touch-ups frequently to combat the oil and shine

OILY SKIN CARE REGIMEN:

If you feel that you have oily skin, try this skin care regimen to help combat some of the side effects like clogged pores and excessive oil production.

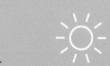

DAYTIME

Cleanse with an **oil cleanser** -> follow by an **oil free moisturizer** w/SPF.

NIGHTTIME

Use an **oil cleanser** again -> double cleanse with a **gel cleanser** if removing makeup -> follow with an **oil free moisturizer.**

MAINTENANCE

Use a **clay mask** 2-3 times a week + exfoliate 3-4 times a week.

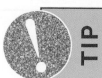

TIP

Don't be afraid to use oil. When you "strip" your skin of the natural oil it produces, your skin goes into overdrive and produces even more oil, which may further clog pores and cause breakouts.

DO I HAVE DRY SKIN?

The characteristics listed below are **most commonly associated with dry skin**. Check off the items on the list that accurately describe your skin to see if this is your skin type. If you check most of the boxes, this is most likely your skin type, so **look for products recommended for dry skin** throughout the rest of this book.

YOU MAY HAVE DRY SKIN IF:

- ○ Your skin feels **tight**
- ○ Your skin appears **dull/flat**
- ○ Your skin lacks glow throughout the day
- ○ Your skin constantly feels the need for more hydration
- ○ Your makeup gets "sucked in" when applied and throughout the day
- ○ You wake up with dryness

DRY SKIN CARE REGIMEN:

If you feel that you have dry skin, try this skin care regimen to help combat some of the side effects like tightness and dryness, and work to rehydrate your skin.

DAYTIME
Use a **milk cleanser**, then apply moisturizer and SPF.

NIGHTTIME
Use an **oil cleanser**, double cleanse again with a **milk cleanser** if removing makeup, then follow with a facial **oil** and **emollient** moisturizer.

MAINTENANCE
Do a **hydration mask** 1-3 times a week and exfoliation 2-3 times a week.

TIP *Keep an alcohol-free **hydrating spray** handy and use it liberally throughout the day to keep dry skin looking dewy and healthy.*

DO I HAVE SENSITIVE SKIN?

The characteristics listed below are **most commonly associated with sensitive skin**. Check off the items on the list that accurately describe your skin to see if this is your skin type. If you check most of the boxes, this is most likely your skin type, so **look for products recommended for sensitive skin** throughout the rest of this book.

YOU MAY HAVE SENSITIVE SKIN IF:

- ◯ Your skin is oftentimes **red or pink**
- ◯ Your skin feels **irritated or rash-like**
- ◯ Your skin quickly **reacts** to new, unfamiliar products
- ◯ You have used or have been told to use a color correction product

SENSITIVE SKIN CARE REGIMEN:

If you feel that you have sensitive skin, try this skin care regimen with products that won't irritate your skin to help combat redness and irritation.

DAYTIME

Use a **mild cleanser** in the morning followed by a **fragrance free** and calming moisturizer and SPF.

NIGHTTIME

Use the exact same cleanser and moisturizer as long as they do not irritate you.

MAINTENANCE

Use a **calming mask** 2-3 times a week use and only exfoliate weekly with a mild manual exfoliant such as something containing **jojoba beads.**

TIP

Use less variation in your products. Let your skin get used to a product and stick with it as much as possible.

DO I HAVE
AGING SKIN?

The characteristics listed below are **most commonly associated with aging skin**. Check off the items on the list that accurately describe your skin to see if this is your skin type. If you check most of the boxes, this is most likely your skin type, so **look for products recommended for aging skin** throughout the rest of this book.

YOU MAY HAVE AGING SKIN IF:

- ◯ There are **fine lines and wrinkles** around your eyes, mouth, and forehead
- ◯ Your skin is starting to **lose elasticity** and firmness
- ◯ You have **dry skin**
- ◯ Makeup seems to gather in lines and wrinkles

AGING SKIN CARE REGIMEN:

If your skin is beginning to show signs of aging, try this skin care regimen to help combat dry skin and some of the other factors that affect the appearance of aging skin.

DAYTIME

Use an **oil cleanser** in the morning followed by an **anti aging** oil, moisturizer and spf.

NIGHTTIME

Use an **oil cleanser** followed by **milk cleanser** if removing makeup, **anti aging serum**, oil and moisturizer.

MAINTENANCE

Use an **anti-aging** and/or hydration mask 2-3 times a week. Exfoliate 2-4 times a week.

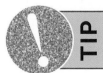

TIP

Exfoliate often. As we age, cell turnover slows down so exfoliation helps speed it back up. Don't forget to moisturize afterwards.

DO I HAVE
COMBINATION SKIN?

The characteristics listed below are **most commonly associated with combination skin**. Check off the items on the list that accurately describe your skin to see if this is your skin type. If you check most of the boxes, this is most likely your skin type, so **look for products recommended for combination skin** throughout the rest of this book.

YOU MAY HAVE COMBINATION SKIN IF:

- ○ Your skin **feels tight** or dry in some places while other parts feel or look oily
- ○ You have visible, **large pores**
- ○ Your makeup application seems uneven
- ○ Makeup slips or slides off in places, usually the T-zone (nose, chin, and forehead)

COMBINATION SKIN CARE REGIMEN:

Combination skin can be tricky. Try this skin care regimen to combat the side effects of dryness and oiliness to even out your complexion.

DAYTIME
Use an **oil cleanser** in the morning followed by an **oil free moisturizer** and/or **mattefying moisturizer** in the oily areas and spf.

NIGHTTIME
Use an **oil cleanser** followed by a **gel cleanser** if removing makeup, a **facial oil** and nourishing moisturizer.

MAINTENANCE
Exfoliate 2-3 times weekly, treat oily areas with a clay mask 2-3 times a week and dry areas with a hydration mask 2-4 times a week.

MAKEUP TOOLS

TALK COLOR TO ME

LEARN IT. LOVE IT. THE BEST TOOL.

The color wheel is something that artists of all mediums use, reference, and memorize! If you have a warm skin tone but wear makeup with cool undertones or vice versa, your makeup may appear ashy and unflattering. **Knowing which colors suit and compliment your skin tone, your eyes, and even your hair, will elevate your makeup game in ways you could never have imagined.** Bookmark this page. Heck, tear it out and frame it! You'll be referencing this page throughout the book!

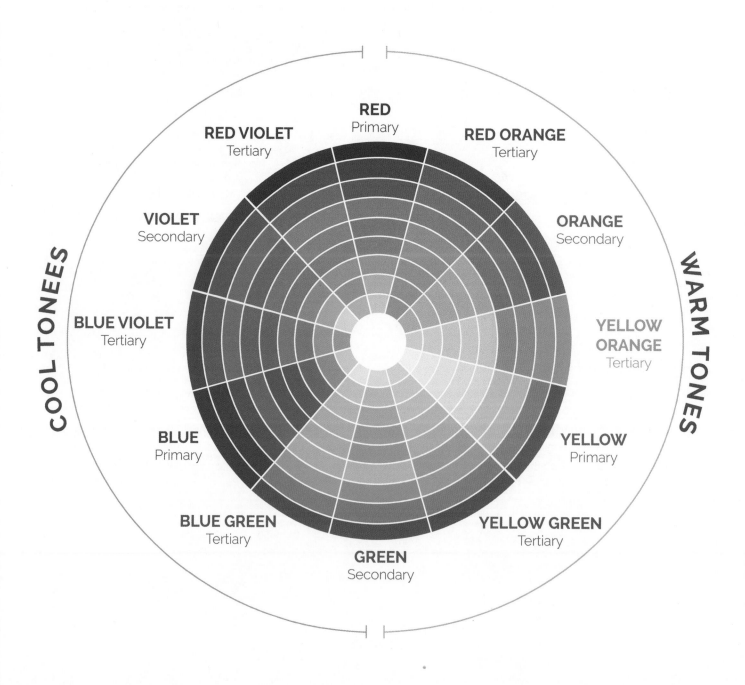

ESSENTIAL TOOLS

Rome wasn't built in a day! Neither was a makeup artist's brush collection! My brushes are hands down the most valuable products in my makeup kit. Why? Not only do they cost the most (an investment I've made over decades) but they also make beautiful makeup possible! With the right tools (not necessarily the most expensive ones), you can make any brand of makeup look like a million bucks.

The graphic below shows the most common and widely available makeup tools, but this is not an all-inclusive list of brushes! By no means do you need to run out and purchase all of these items but at least you'll recognize these tools when you are shopping and can pick up the correct ones when you need or are ready to use them.

STIPPLING BRUSH
Perfect for buffing liquid, cream, or mousse foundation. Use small, circular strokes to blend.

FOUNDATION BRUSH
Use this flat brush to apply liquid foundation by swiping back and forth until blended.

POWDER BRUSH
A large, fluffy brush perfect for applying powder over the top of foundation.

FAN BRUSH
This thin, flat brush is great for applying highlighter and lightly dusting off any excess product that may have fallen out.

BLUSH BRUSH
A medium sized brush perfect for applying and blending blush and bronzer.

ANGLED CHEEK BRUSH
This slanted brush is ideal for a various applications, such as blush, bronzer and contouring.

LIP BRUSH
Use this small, flat brush to apply lipstick and glosses with precision.

EYE SHADOW BRUSH
Flat brushes that come in large and small sizes, perfect for applying eyeshadow on the lid.

CREASE BRUSH
The slight angle of this brush helps get in the crease of the eyelid to easily blend shadow.

BLENDING BRUSH
This small, fluffy brush is ideal for blending different shadow colors for a more natural look.

EYELINER BRUSH
Use an angled or straight brush to get a perfect eyeliner application or to fill in brows.

EYEBROW BRUSH
The eyebrow comb and spoolie are used to brush and groom brows to make them appear fuller.

BEAUTY SPONGE
This bulb-shaped sponge is best used dampened. Pat and blend liquid foundation, concealer, blush, and highlighter.

KABUKI BRUSH
Use this short, stubby brush to buff on powder foundation in small circular motions. Can use lightly to apply blush or bronzer.

TOOLS EXPLAINED

SYNTHETIC VS. NATURAL HAIR BRUSHES

Synthetic brushes generally work/blend well with cream products. Natural hair brushes generally work/blend well with powder products. However, as you experiment and find which brushes you like and love, you'll slowly discover that the rules of brushes and makeup are meant to be broken!

Professional makeup artists are always breaking the rules, using brushes marketed for one purpose and repurposing them for a different one! Start small with your brush collection. Avoid purchasing "sets" if you are new to the makeup game and feel extremely overwhelmed by shopping for brushes. Instead, get comfortable with a few brushes at a time and you'll slowly build an amazing collection that won't overwhelm or intimidate you!

TIP

One theme you'll find throughout this book is to do your own research! Animal and environment lovers generally lean towards building a fully synthetic brush kit! However, the glues and chemicals and components that compose synthetic brushes may contain animal products and are not necessarily better for the environment. Natural hair brushes could be hand-made from ethically trimmed animal hairs. It's really your job to do the research and not take everything at face value!

BEAUTY SPONGES

Beauty sponges have come a long way in the last few decades! The shape, design, and even the texture has improved the application of makeup in so many ways! Keep these sponges clean (which we will get to in the next section) and they'll serve you well for plenty of time to come.

VELOUR PUFFS

Velour puffs have been around forever! They are soft, they don't disturb makeup, and they are versatile for powder applications and powdering your face throughout the day! You should at least have one clean puff sitting around -- get a good one and you can throw it in the wash!

FINGERTIPS

When I say fingertips, I always mean clean fingertips. Your hands should always be freshly washed (at a minimum sanitized) when using your fingers to apply makeup. When using multiple makeup products, you'll probably have to wash your hands several times! This is my preferred method of application for most cream products!

TIP

Most face makeup can be applied with your fingers or a synthetic face brush. A blush brush can double as a bronzer brush, a highlighter brush, and even a "contour" brush, should that be your thing! Oftentimes, I sweep whatever is left on my blush/ bronzer brush across my eyes and call it a day! Invest in a good beauty sponge and a few quality brushes, that's all you need for a flawless daytime makeup look.

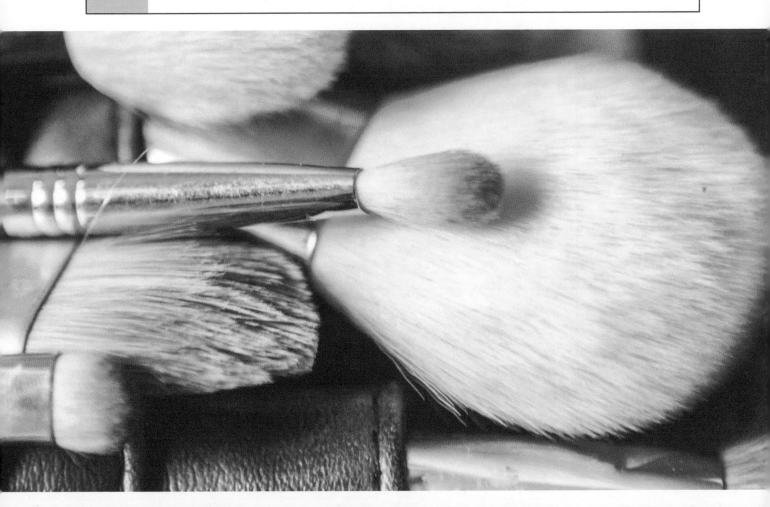

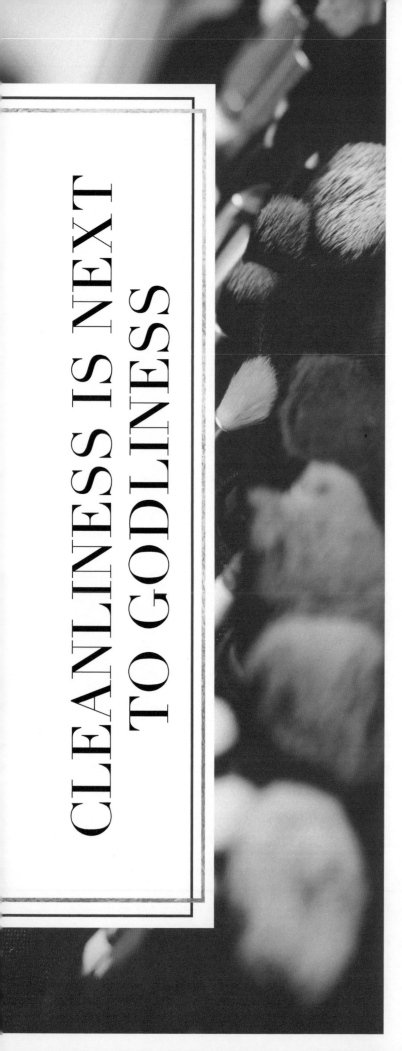

CLEANLINESS IS NEXT TO GODLINESS

HOW TO CLEAN YOUR BRUSHES

You want to take care of your brushes so that they'll last you at least half a lifetime -- so using gentle, mild soaps that still clean well is the route you want to go. Avoid artificial fragrances and perfumes, alcohol, and other harsh chemicals.

BRUSH SOAPS OR BABY SHAMPOO?

There are so many different brush cleansers on the market and at all price points! Sometimes the sheer number of choices makes actually washing your brushes daunting. So either bite the bullet and buy a brush soap or get yourself a bottle of fragrance free baby shampoo. I washed my personal brushes for decades with baby shampoo because it was convenient to find in stores, inexpensive, and did the job. Even in a pinch, I'll still turn to baby shampoo if I don't have a professional brush cleaner around.

FREQUENCY

Wash your brushes monthly, if not more. Don't "share" brushes without fully cleaning them between uses. Never share mascara. Never share lipstick or lipgloss. Never put testers or demos from anything at beauty counters onto your face!

ALCOHOL

70% Isopropyl Alcohol spray is great for sanitizing your powder cosmetics. Less than 70% evaporates too quickly; more than 70% doesn't fully sanitize. Generously spritz the top coat of your powder cosmetics, let it air out for a minute or two, and voila! Your powders are clean.

DOUBLE DIPPING

For cream products or products that are "dunked" in and out -- be careful! Concealer wands when placed on top of a zit takes all that bacteria and contaminates the wand as well as the entire jar. To keep your cream products clean, use a stainless steel spatula and scrape product onto the back of your non-writing hand or apply to a stainless steel makeup plate. If you are prone to breakouts, applying dirty makeup with dirty brushes is not going to help.

MAKEUP

RULES OF THUMB

#1 | PRACTICE MAKES PERFECT!

Sure, you can watch makeup videos all day long and scroll through inspirational and aspirational makeup images, but not until you know your skin type, skin tone, and really start practicing (knowing that you can wash all the makeup off), can you truly become your own makeup artist.

#2 | ALWAYS APPLY MAKEUP TO A CLEAN, FRESHLY MOISTURIZED FACE.

Always. When going from day to night, you may need to spritz a refreshing facial toner or water onto the face before "adding" more makeup. If you apply makeup to an un-moisturized face, you are only asking for trouble!

#3 | LESS IS MORE.

Less makeup is always more. Period.
You don't have to wear a lot of makeup to wear makeup.

#4 | HAVE FUN!

Makeup should be fun. It should be an artistic expression of yourself, whatever that means to you. If you like to keep it natural for the most part but glam it up every once in awhile, great! If you are full glam all day everyday but decide to go makeup-less every now and then, great! This book isn't encouraging you to wear or not wear makeup. This book is encouraging you to learn how to wear makeup, so that you can when you want to!

FACE MAKEUP

FALL IN LOVE WITH YOUR FACE

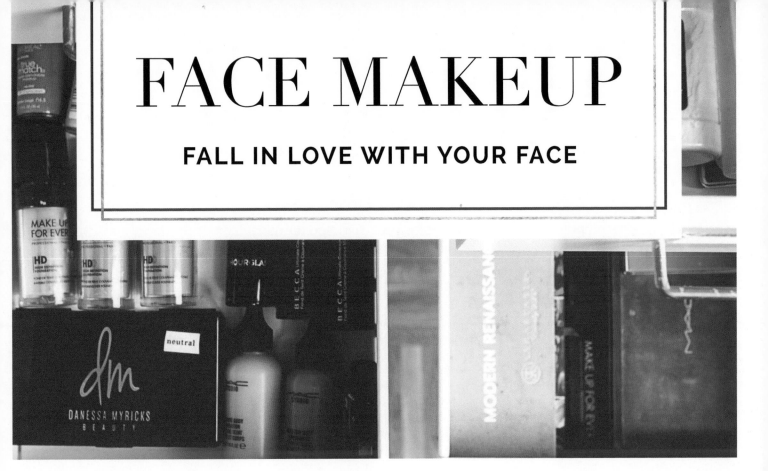

Now that you've identified your skin type, the next step is identifying skin tone. Once you know those two things you are officially ready to apply makeup on your face. Upon completion of this section, you'll have a better understanding of what products and colors will work best for your skin tone, skin type, and also personal preferences. You'll be able to confidently shop for makeup, either solo without assistance or you'll be able to ask pointed questions to sales people and be shown products you know will work for you!

IMPORTANT TO NOTE:

When I use the word foundation in this book, I am referring to any/all types of foundations I list out in the next few pages. Foundation can be a tinted moisturizer or a balm; it can be your CC cream or your mineral powder you apply with a sponge.

WHAT IS YOUR UNDERTONE?

Certain skin tones are prone to skin types however, be aware of these generalizations. Skin tone is an objective and holistic look at the color your skin. **Spoiler alert!** Our skin tone varies (lighter and darker in some places) and of course, our skin tone varies by season and sometimes even between brands.

COOL

○ If your skin has pink, red, or blueish undertones

○ You **burn easily** in the sun

○ You look best in **silver jewelry**

You probably have a **cool** skin tone.

WARM

○ If you have yellow or golden-olive undertones to your skin

○ You **tan easily** in the sun

○ You look best in **gold jewelry**

You probably have a **warm** skin tone.

NEUTRAL

○ If you have both red/pink and golden/yellow undertones

○ You can't tell the undertone

○ You can pull off mixed metals

You probably have a **neutral** skin tone.

RESOURCE *Terri Tomlinson has developed a flesh toned color wheel that **really** helps you hone in on your skin tone and undertone! She'd say there's no such thing as having neutral skin!*

TIP *You can generally warm up neutral foundations with bronzers and blushes, but it is hard to cool down a neutral foundation.*

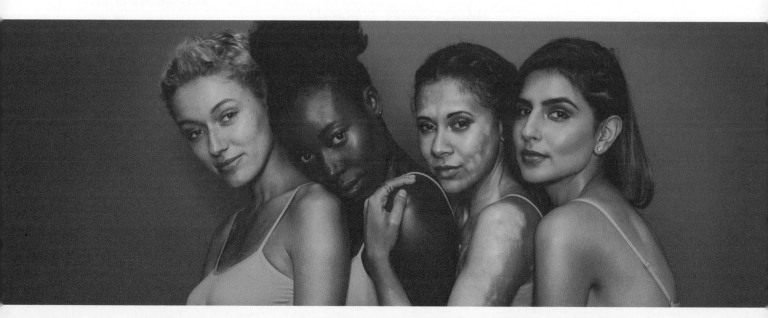

KNOW THY SKIN TONE

Now that you know your undertone and skin type, you can learn how to match your skin tone to makeup. Knowing your skin tone allows you to match makeup colors and hues that compliment you and are flattering. This is especially important when it comes to foundation and concealer. **You must match your skin tone to the makeup, and not the other way around.** *(This is *not* representative of all the gorgeous skin tones).*

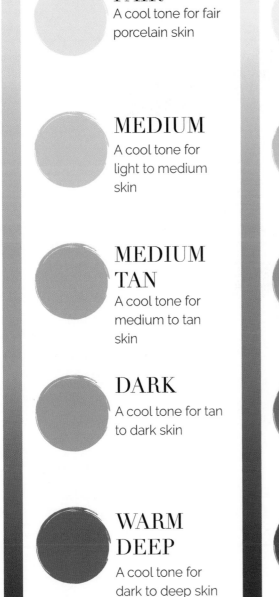
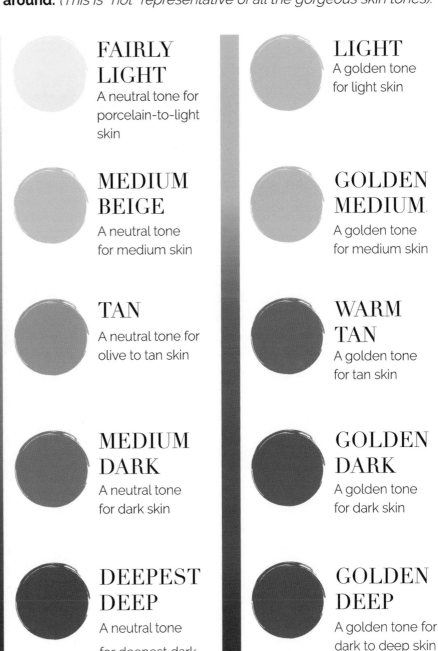

FAIR
A cool tone for fair porcelain skin

FAIRLY LIGHT
A neutral tone for porcelain-to-light skin

LIGHT
A golden tone for light skin

MEDIUM
A cool tone for light to medium skin

MEDIUM BEIGE
A neutral tone for medium skin

GOLDEN MEDIUM
A golden tone for medium skin

MEDIUM TAN
A cool tone for medium to tan skin

TAN
A neutral tone for olive to tan skin

WARM TAN
A golden tone for tan skin

DARK
A cool tone for tan to dark skin

MEDIUM DARK
A neutral tone for dark skin

GOLDEN DARK
A golden tone for dark skin

WARM DEEP
A cool tone for dark to deep skin

DEEPEST DEEP
A neutral tone for deepest dark

GOLDEN DEEP
A golden tone for dark to deep skin

TIP

Gone are the days where you can't find a match. Cosmetic companies (especially high end and luxury brands) have become much better about being inclusive of all skin tones.

SKIN PRIMERS

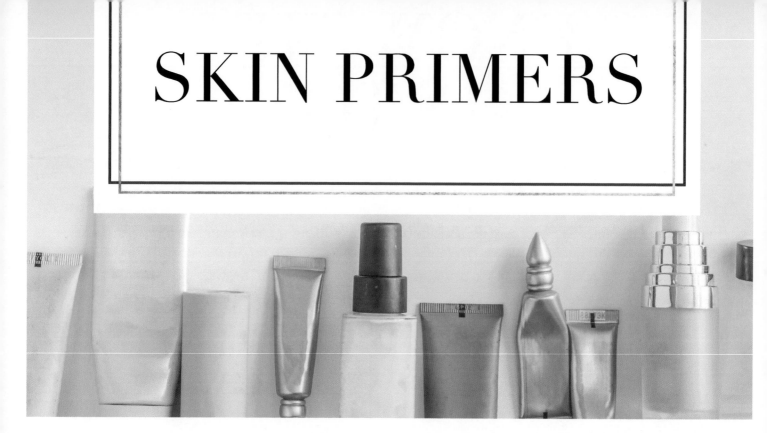

Primers work to smooth out your face and can also help your makeup stay in place all day long (they act like a 'glue' for foundation). If you suffer from acne, acne scarring, or discoloration, primers can also even out your skin tone and texture!

Primers are not in my "everyday" makeup category and most professional makeup artists skip the primer (because good skin care and skin prep is the best primer!) however, primers are nice to have on hand!

Choosing the right primer means knowing your skin type and choosing a product meant to specifically help your most common skin issues.

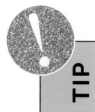

TIP

Make sure that the foundation you choose to wear over or mix in with your primer is not in opposition to it, e.g. mixing an oil-free primer with a foundation that has silicone in it and vice versa. Oil and water don't mix!

TYPES OF PRIMERS

There are several different types of primers, all of which generally serve a different purpose. Two of the most common categories are water-based or oil-free primers and silicone-based primers. They can be in liquid, cream, serum, and powder form. Good skin care generally replaces the need for a primer however, primers have great utility in smoothing out skin texture, evening out skin tone, and extending the wear of makeup throughout the day.

OIL FREE PRIMERS

Oil free primers are great for those with **oily or combination skin**. Although you shouldn't need primer after prepping your skin for makeup -- applying an oil free primer in the oily zones can help the longevity of your makeup application. Look for a mattefying formula when shopping for an oil free primer!

CHARACTERISTICS

- Does not add excess oils to face
- May feel tacky on skin, especially if applied on non-oily areas (combination skin)
- Silicone free!

PROS

- May minimize the appearance of pores
- Reduces shine
- Many oil free primers are also water-based! Great for adding healthy moisture (not more oils) to your face

SILICONE BASED PRIMERS

Silicone based primers are great for dry or normal to dry skin and can do a beautiful job of smoothing out textured skin.

CHARACTERISTICS

- May give skin a soft velvet texture
- Tinted silicone primers may also help even out skin tone
- Can slide off of "oily" patches or oily skin

PROS

- Fill fine lines and wrinkles
- Creates a blurring effect
- Flexible wear on skin

HOW TO APPLY PRIMER

 Unless you have extremely oily skin and/or fingertips, it's best to apply primer with your fingers!

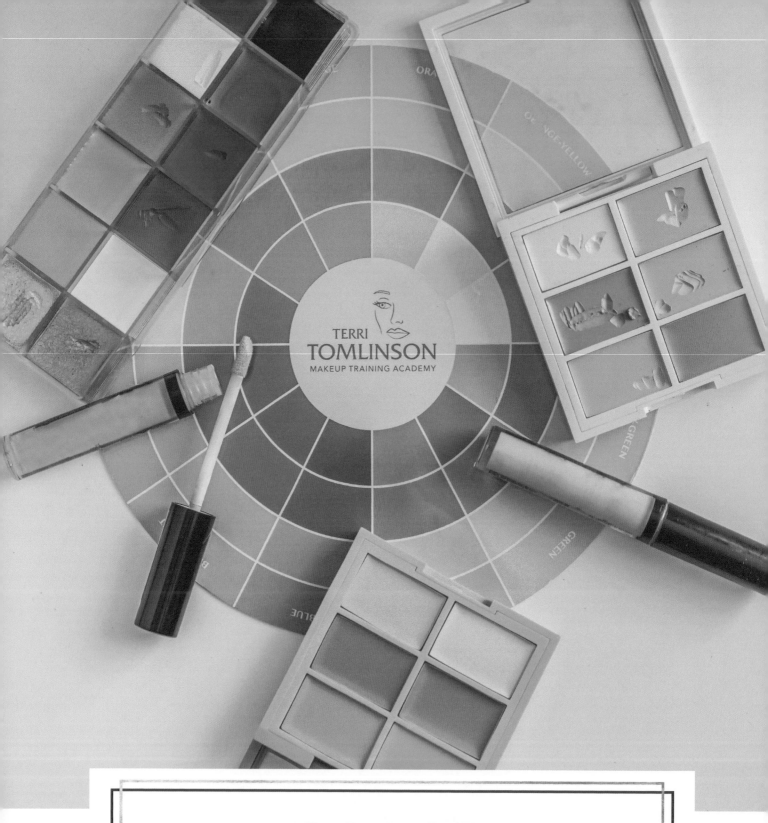

COLOR CORRECTION

COLOR CORRECTORS

If you have small or large areas of redness, darkness, melasma, etc. color correctors can be your best friend! By referring to the color wheel and the graphic below, you can see which colors cancel out which colors.

Most of the time, good skincare, a bit of color correcting primer, and good foundation can even out areas of pigmentation on the face. If not, color correcting "sticks" or concealer (generally sold in liquid and cream formulas), can aid in neutralizing these areas.

Color correcting is an art and takes time to master. When you are watching a makeup tutorial online, it may look extremely effortless but that is because these artists are in bright studio lights, so they'll tend to apply more. You also cannot see the "pressure" they are applying with! Also, you may or may not see video breaks or edits from start to finish. **Be careful when imitating color correction!**

GREEN CANCELS RED	**YELLOW CANCELS PURPLE**
ORANGE CANCELS BLUE	**PURPLE CANCELS BROWN**

 ## DOUBLE DUTY APPLICATION:

This product can pull double duty! *Color correcting primers are amazing at both acting as a primer as well as neutralizing larger areas of pigmentation. For example, a green primer is great for evening out redness on the skin without adding more color correcting products.*

COLOR CORRECTORS
IN ACTION

BEFORE

AFTER

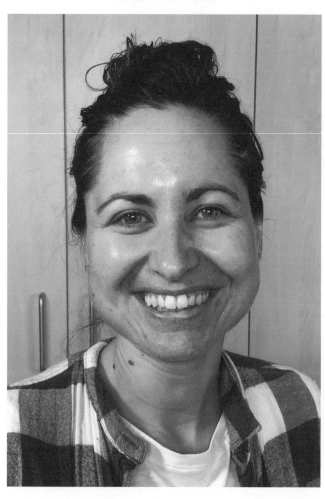

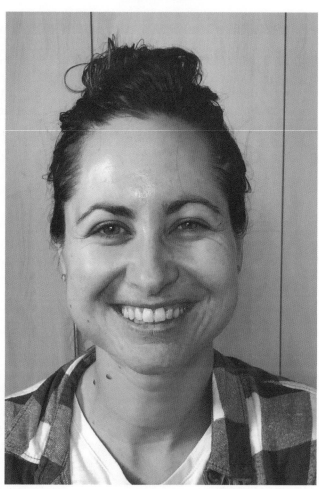

Using color correctors can make a huge difference in the appearance of your skin and creates a "blank slate" for your makeup application.

These before and after photos show the difference that a single application of color correcting primer can produce. In this application, the primer was green canceling out the red undertones in her skin.

Consult your dermatologist and/or an esthetician to look for underlying causes of skin redness or discoloration. Makeup is simply a bandaid to a potentially treatable underlying skin discoloration.

FOUNDATION

THE FUNDAMENTALS

Foundation is a product that evens out your skin tone -- and when worn alone, can make you look like a ghost (because we have so many other tones in our faces). So if you plan on wearing foundation, plan on at least wearing blush or bronzer. Don't worry, we'll get to that in the next few chapters.

FOUNDATION BASICS

For now, let's talk about the basics of foundation. First, it's important to know that foundation has come a long way since the days of cakey, thick, pore-clogging formulas -- although they still exist!

Today's technology has created lightweight, full coverage foundations that don't feel or look heavy on the skin, with proper application (hello HD, 4K, 5K television!) and the great news is that these foundations are available at all price points! If you've been avoiding wearing foundation, now is the time to give it another chance!

This is where preference comes in. Maybe you like a sheer layer with amazing skincare benefits, a full coverage foundation, or something in between. As your skin type or preferences change, so should your foundation!

WHAT COMES FIRST?
CONCEALER OR FOUNDATION?

The general rule of thumb is this - If you are applying powder foundation, then you must use concealers and/or correctors first! If you are applying liquid/cream foundations, then you'd use concealers after!

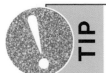

TIP

You may be multi-tonal and need to use more than one foundation, or your tone may change seasonally! That's totally normal. Consider blending your winter & summer foundation to bridge fall & spring. A good match is always in style!

CHOOSING THE RIGHT FOUNDATION

There are a lot of different foundation formulas out there, and it can be a little overwhelming. Knowing the pros and cons of different foundations will help you find the right formula for you.

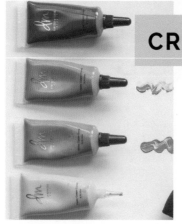

CREAM FOUNDATION

Cream foundation is used by a lot of professional working makeup artists on film, television, stage, and print. Cream foundations are extremely full coverage, but can be sheered out with moisturizers, thinners, or oils for lightweight wear.

- You might like cream foundations if you prefer a full coverage look.
- Cream concealers most often are sold in compacts, pots, or palettes.
- Cream foundations can look cakey, fast!
- Cream foundations are generally good for all skin types -- but quality skin prep is required if you want your cream foundation to look amazing all day!

Cream foundations are best applied with a synthethic foundation brush, warmed up on the back of your hand or spatula.

LIQUID FOUNDATION

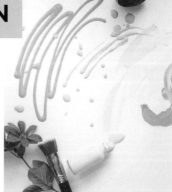

Liquid foundations are mixable, buildable and flexible! They come out of pumps or bottles and can be custom blended quickly and easily.

- Avoid SPF in your liquid foundations if you are worried about flashback! Not all, but some liquid foundations are notorious for flashback aka shiny face in photos with flash photography.

Liquid foundations can be applied in many ways: fingers, beauty sponges, and/or foundation brushes. I prefer applying with my fingers and then pressing in with a sponge to distribute everything evenly!

WITHOUT
FOUNDATION

WITH
FOUNDATION

LAYING
FOUNDATIONS

A great foundation application is an essential building block
for your look! It evens the skin tone and creates a clean
slate for all the fun ahead!

CONCEALER

CONCEALER 101

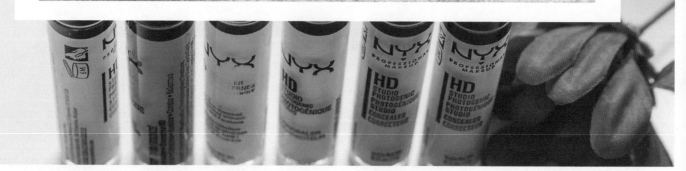

Unlike correctors, concealers are generally used in **your exact skin shade or one shade lighter and with a touch of yellow** (to correct the general dark purple under the eye). Concealers generally come in tube, stick, or cream form.

There's two schools of thought around when you should apply concealer. Some say before foundation and some insist it's best after foundation. Applying after foundation guarantees your concealer won't go to waste, but it may take more time to blend it out. Apply before if you are in a hurry, apply after for a more precise application!

CHOOSING THE RIGHT CONCEALER

The number one problem I see with concealer is overuse and misuse.

A good foundation match with excellent coverage normally negates the need for concealers. If it doesn't, then you should maybe explore some different foundation formulations!

Sometimes, a small amount of concealer may be needed under the eyes or on top of a stubborn pimple, or even in the corners of the eye for brightening. Just because the whole world is seemingly dousing their faces in concealer doesn't mean you should. Concealer is essentially concentrated foundation and should be used sparingly and with caution.

LIQUID OR CREAM?

WHICH SHOULD YOU USE?

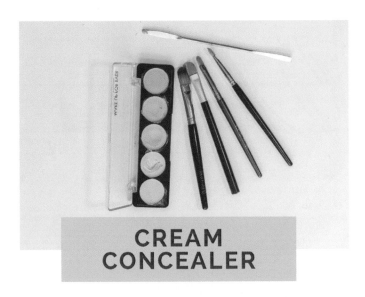

CREAM CONCEALER

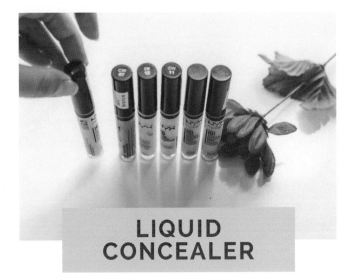

LIQUID CONCEALER

Like cream foundation, cream concealer is extremely highly pigmented and is best used for spot correction (e.g. the huge zit that popped up overnight). You wouldn't want to use cream concealers in large areas.

Remember, concealer does not make the texture disappear, just evens out the color.

- Typically offers the most coverage
- Harder to work with; warm up on back of hand/palette before applying
- Best used for spot concealing
- Good for tattoo coverup (alcohol based)
- Tends to dry out quickly in packaging, buying a small size is better as to not waste product

Liquid concealer is accessible, comes in nearly every shade under the sun, and is also what you see people painting their faces with all over the internet!

While watching people sculpt their faces with concealer is mesmerizing, that doesn't mean you should do it yourself.

- More sheer and versatile than cream concealers, better for larger areas
- Easy to use, but hard to keep clean (double dipping)
- Most offer medium coverage
- Not ideal for spot concealing or extensive color correction
- Settles in creases if not set properly

APPLY WITH:

APPLY WITH:

CONCEALER APPLICATION

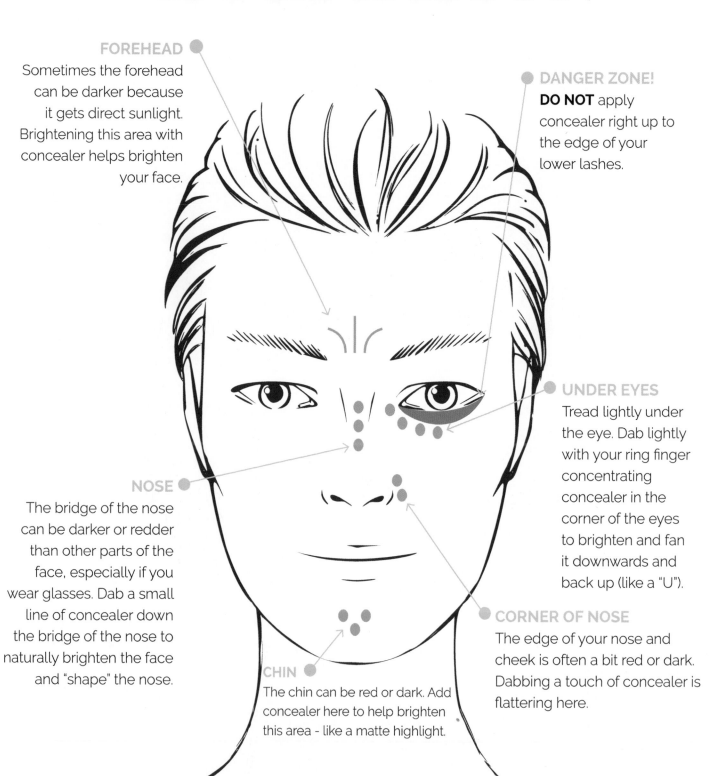

FOREHEAD
Sometimes the forehead can be darker because it gets direct sunlight. Brightening this area with concealer helps brighten your face.

DANGER ZONE!
DO NOT apply concealer right up to the edge of your lower lashes.

UNDER EYES
Tread lightly under the eye. Dab lightly with your ring finger concentrating concealer in the corner of the eyes to brighten and fan it downwards and back up (like a "U").

NOSE
The bridge of the nose can be darker or redder than other parts of the face, especially if you wear glasses. Dab a small line of concealer down the bridge of the nose to naturally brighten the face and "shape" the nose.

CORNER OF NOSE
The edge of your nose and cheek is often a bit red or dark. Dabbing a touch of concealer is flattering here.

CHIN
The chin can be red or dark. Add concealer here to help brighten this area - like a matte highlight.

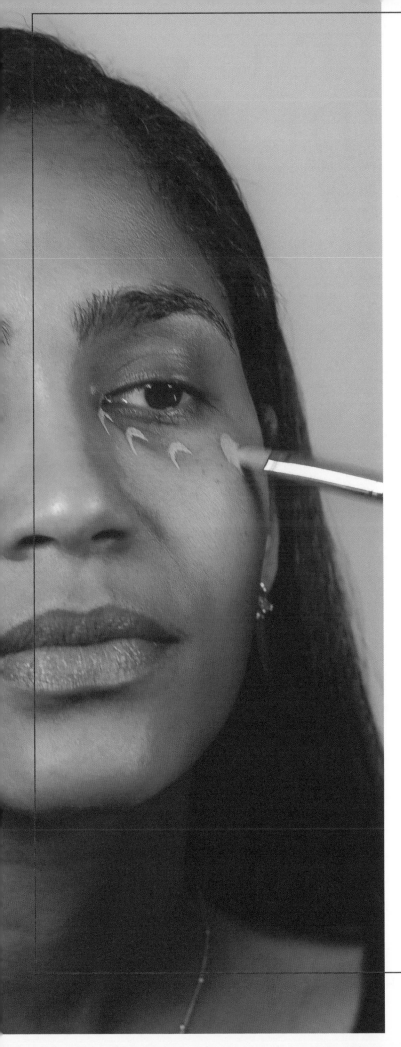

UNDER EYE CONCEALER TIPS

One of the most popular blog posts I wrote was all about undereye concealer. It can be the most frustrating part of makeup application because the delicate under eye area tends to "collect" makeup products and notoriously creases. When applying concealer under the eye you must be mindful to use it strategically and sparingly.

CREASING GOT YOU DOWN?

Using a mattefying eye primer under the eye may help to keep concealer and powders from creasing under the eye.

WRINKLES UNDER THE EYE?

If you have any signs of aging on your skin, you absolutely need to **set your concealer with a small amount of setting powder**. If you don't, your concealer will "crease" over the course of the day. Use a brush or sponge and dust away any excess before applying. You want a setting powder that is finely milled and translucent in color (or skin tone). See next section for more info!

RING FINGER, BEST FINGER!

Your ring finger is the preferred finger for applying concealer, especially under the eye It is so important not to use too much pressure when applying concealer. The little veins under your eyes are easily irritated, which causes them to become discolored (from being tired or pressing too hard on them). Lightly dab and press concealer onto this area so you do not irritate your sensitive under eye area.

SETTING POWDER

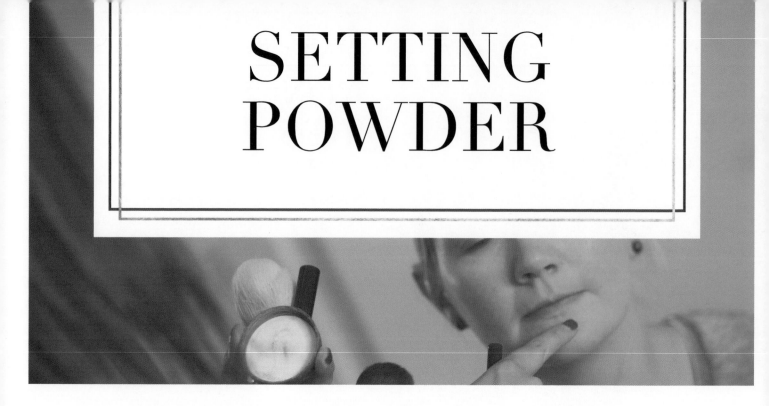

Loose powder is most often used to set foundation and concealer. This is an important step so often skipped by many, but if you don't "set" your foundation and/or concealer with a translucent or flesh toned loose powder, you'll likely suffer from creasing, oiliness, and blotchiness before the day is over. ***You can skip this step if you are using a powder foundation or pressed powder.***

SETTING YOUR FOUNDATION

You can also use your beauty sponge to set your foundation anywhere on the face. You do so by lightly pressing and "rolling" the blender onto the areas of the face you are setting! Make sure to brush off any residual powder with a large fluffy brush.

The fluffy powder puff is always a fun brush to use for an all over set. It's especially great if you aren't using much or any concealer.

Alternatively, you can apply your loose powder with a beauty sponge or smaller powder or kabuki brush. Always make sure to brush off any excess!

SETTING YOUR CONCEALER

Setting your foundation with loose powder is optional, but you should ALWAYS set your concealer. Using a small blending blush or medium face brush is optimal for setting concealer.

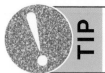 *"Set" your tinted moisturizer if you want more coverage without wearing a full-coverage foundation!*

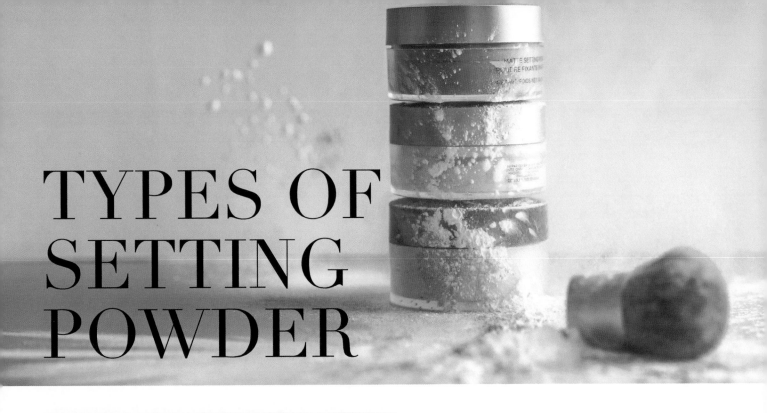

TYPES OF SETTING POWDER

TRANSLUCENT

Translucent powder is finely milled powder that is more or less "see-thru". Translucent powder generally has a hint of pigment in it, so when buying translucent powder, make sure you purchase in the correct shade range (normaly light/medium and medium/dark).

TRANSLUCENT POWDER PROS...

- ○ Helps with oil control
- ○ Sets your foundation application
- ○ Helps blur the appearance of pores

NO-COLOR

No-Color powder is much like translucent powder however, there is no color. Although the powder is white when applied, it sheers out colorlessly. This is a perfect powder for touch ups since it doesn't disturb makeup.

NO-COLOR POWDER PROS...

- ○ Pigment free
- ○ Won't disturb makeup application

FINISHING POWDERS

Finishing powder is another powder that is most often used for theatrical, on-camera, or "bright lights" appearances. Unlike translucent and no-color powder, finishing powder may disturb the makeup with the desired finishing effect (e.g. glowing, mattefying, adding more coverage). These powders can appear incredibly cakey quickly and are not intended for day-to-day use, unless of course your work involves being on a stage or on a set.

PIGMENTED POWDER PROS...

- ○ Great for "on-camera" or stage use
- ○ Comes in a variety of finishing effects
- ○ Provides additional coverage

ABOUT BAKING

Baking has it's roots in the drag theatrical community and grew in popularity with the rise of contouring and strobing. Baking essentially means placing an excessive amount of setting powder onto the face and brushing off the excess after a bit of time passes, most commonly used under the eyes and along the jawline. In the drag community, this really helped the performers have more pronounced face shapes. This is still a technique used often in the theatrical community but for day-to-day application, baking generally appears extremely heavy and is often times unnecessary (especially under the eyes!)

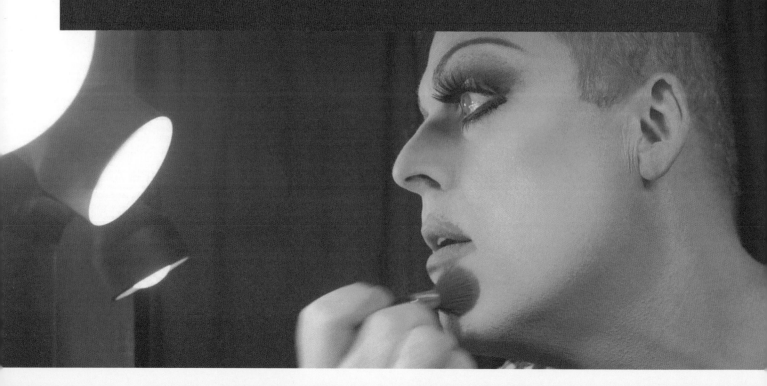

SETTING POWDER APPLICATION

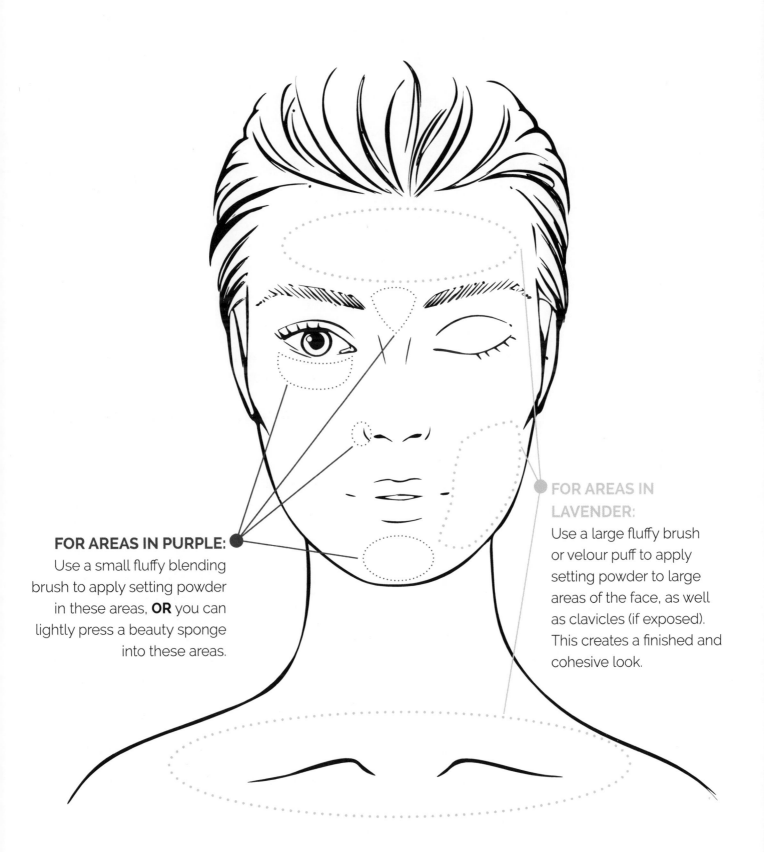

FOR AREAS IN PURPLE:
Use a small fluffy blending brush to apply setting powder in these areas, **OR** you can lightly press a beauty sponge into these areas.

FOR AREAS IN LAVENDER:
Use a large fluffy brush or velour puff to apply setting powder to large areas of the face, as well as clavicles (if exposed). This creates a finished and cohesive look.

UNDERSTANDING YOUR FACE SHAPE

We all have different body types and we also have different face shapes. **Falling in love with your face shape is one of the most important things you can do**, especially when it comes to makeup. When you become deeply familiar with your face shape, you'll know exactly where to apply blush, bronzer, and highlighter! If you are lost, find a celebrity with your face shape and see where/how they apply blush, bronzer, and highlighter!

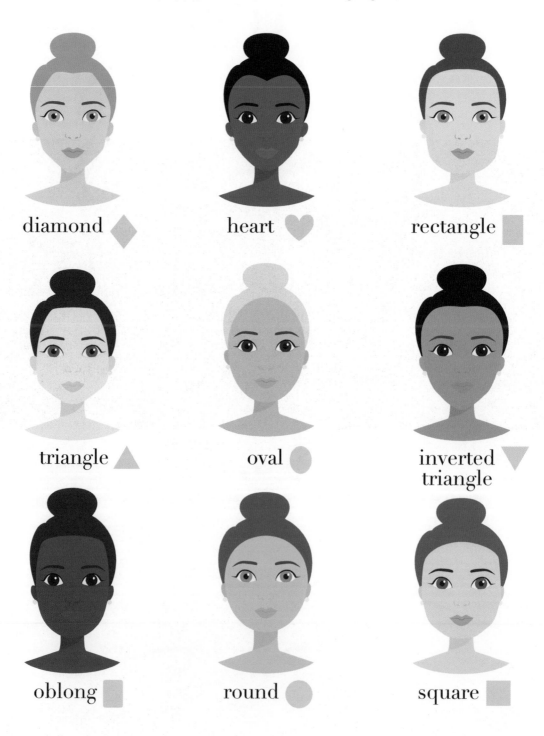

diamond ◆   heart ♥   rectangle ▮

triangle ▲   oval ⬭   inverted triangle ▼

oblong ▮   round ●   square ▮

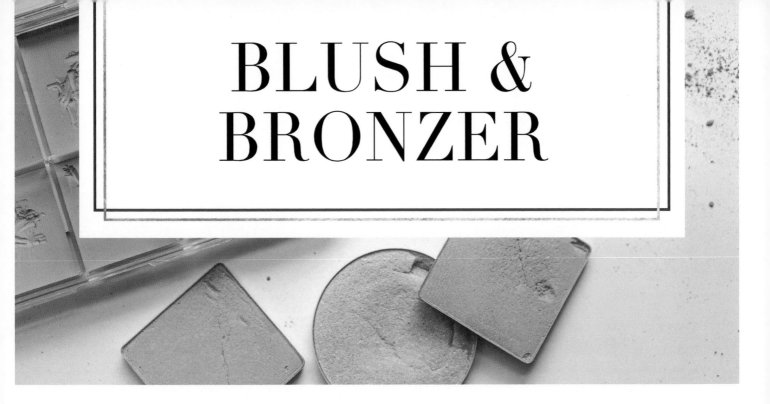

BLUSH &
BRONZER

You've finally found a perfect foundation match, you've evened out your skin tone with foundation, concealed all those little worries away, and now you are left looking in the mirror a little bit like a ghost!

Well, that's because you sort of are!

This is the part of the makeup application where you can actually start having some real fun with color! This is also the part of the makeup application personal preferences and a working knowledge of the color wheel really matter. Having the wrong color blush in your makeup bag can be detrimental and can age you 10 years in 10 seconds!

In this section you'll learn about how/why/when/where to apply blush, bronzer, and highlighter. I'll discuss quickly what this fad of "contouring" is all about. You deserve the truth, the whole truth, and nothing but the truth, okay?

IT'S BLUSH TIME!

BLUSH

IT'S OKAY TO BLUSH WITH ME

Blush is seriously one of those products (like a red lipstick) that freaks people out. So many choices to pick from and fears of looking straight up like a clown post-application -- most people bow out of makeup altogether because they've managed to figure out how to wear their foundation but can't figure out blush, and they can't figure out why they look terrible in pictures... You can see where I'm going here.

Fear not, my friend. Blush can be (and should be) one of your besties! Why? Because it's something you already have! Naturally!

HOW TO PICK OUT THE RIGHT BLUSH COLOR FOR YOU

Look in the mirror before you put on makeup. Pinch your cheeks if you can't see what color you are! For those of you who want to keep it really natural, pick a color blush that most closely resembles your natural blush color and has your same undertone (remember that?).

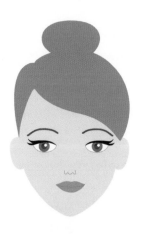

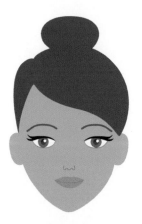

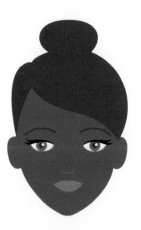

COOL TONES
If your skin has cool tones, find a pink shade with blue or purple undertones.

NEUTRAL TONES
Neutrals can be tricky. I generally recommend mauve, but play around to find what works best.

WARM TONES
If your skin has warm tones, find a blush with yellow or coral undertones.

Remember, fair skin doesn't always mean cool, and dark skin doesn't always mean warm!

TYPES OF BLUSH

CREAM & LIQUID BLUSH

Cream and liquid blushes are hands down some of my favorite products of all time! They come in so many different colors and formulations, the sky is truly the limit.

CREAM & LIQUID BLUSH WILL...

- ◯ Blend naturally into your skin
- ◯ Last longer than powder
- ◯ Work on a variety of skin types

CREAM & LIQUID BLUSH PROS...

- ◯ Great for mature skin
- ◯ Easy to blend
- ◯ Act as a great base for powders

DOUBLE DUTY APPLICATION:

This product can pull double duty! *Your cream blush can be swept onto the eyelids for a natural flush of color as well as onto the lips. You can create a gorgeous monochromatic look with cream blushes!*

HOW TO APPLY CREAM BLUSH

Cream blushes are best applied directly onto skin with fingertips and blended naturally into skin.

If you have oily fingertips, try using a flat or small kabuki synthetic brush, blending in with the fingers or buffing with a clean sponge or brush.

POWDER BLUSH

Unlike cream/liquid blushes, powder blushes can offer amazing little bursts of color, quickly and relatively effortlessly. When you use a blush with shimmer, you can add a bit of extra glow and skip the highlighter! While powder blushes don't last as long as creams do, when applied properly they can quickly intensify your look and add dimension to the face.

POWDER BLUSH WILL...

- ○ Create a burst of color on the face
- ○ Add dimension to the face
- ○ Work in place of a highlighter if you use a shimmer blush.

POWDER BLUSH PROS...

- ○ Easy application
- ○ Great for oily skin types
- ○ When applied on top of cream blush, it can extend the longevity of the color.

HOW TO APPLY POWDER BLUSH

 I prefer to use a natural hair blush brush to apply blush. There are lots of different sizes and shapes of blush brushes out there. You need to find a brush that is proportionate to the apples of your cheeks. If you buy a blush brush that's too big or too small, your powder blush will not apply in a flattering way.

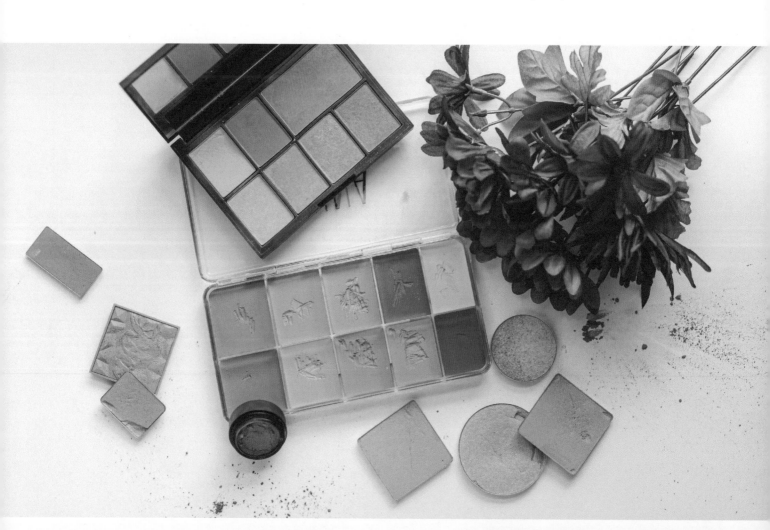

BLUSH APPLICATION

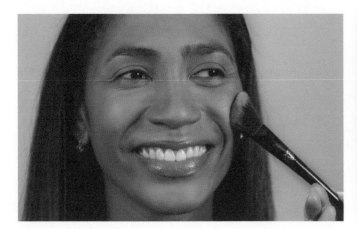 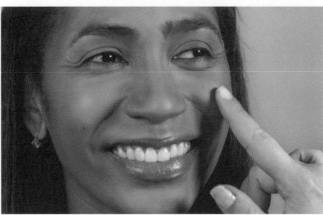

Blush should not extend past an invisible line drawn down the center of your eye when you are looking forward.

CONCENTRATE COLOR ON THE APPLES OF YOUR CHEEKS!
The #1 rule for knowing where to apply blush (regardless of face shape) is to *smile*, find the apples of the cheeks and apply there. Blend color up along the cheekbone.

Blush should go on or above the cheekbones and should not extend below the hollow of your cheeks.

Page 55

WITHOUT
BLUSH

WITH
BLUSH

BLUSHING
BEAUTY

Adding a bit of blush to your look helps to brighten your
entire face. See the difference in the two sides of the face
with and without blush?

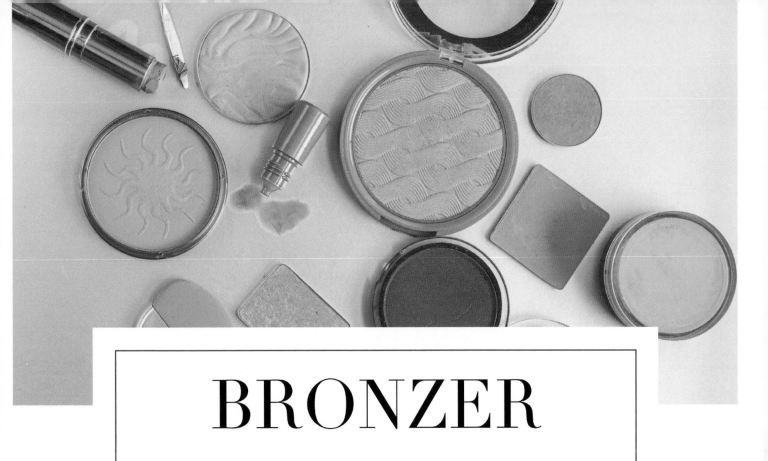

BRONZER

Where blush adds that natural flush back to your skin… bronzer adds that tan!

Bronzers, when applied correctly, can add an extra bit of dimension to the face that blush and highlighter can't achieve. Bronzers are one of my favorite products to use in the summer. A little bit of tinted moisturizer, a touch of bronzer applied underneath the apples of the cheek and swept across the nose and eyes, with a good coat of mascara and you'll have a fresh summer face of makeup in no time!

Unlike eyeshadows and blushes, once you find your perfect bronzer color, you'll likely end up sticking with it for years to come!

DOUBLE DUTY APPLICATION:

This product can pull double duty! *Matte bronzers can be used as a contour powder, especially if you bought a shade too dark or if it's winter and your skin is a shade or two lighter than your summer skin. Once summer rolls around, it can be used as a bronzer again! You can also use bronzers as a matte crease color for your eyes!*

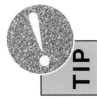

Because bronzers tend to be "warm toned" colors, if you are fair or cool toned, applying the wrong color bronzer may appear orange on the skin! Shopping for neutral bronzers is best!

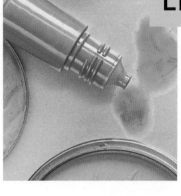

LIQUID BRONZER
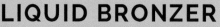

- Liquid bronzers are super versatile products! They can be applied under the foundation to add natural dimension as well as on top of foundation.
- They generally sheer out quite a bit with good blending techniques and are easily to build up - so start off with a small amount and add more should you want to intensify the look.

 HOW TO APPLY: My favorite way to apply liquid bronzers are with my fingers. Then, I use either a beauty sponge to really press and blend it into the skin to look natural.

CREAM BRONZER

- Like liquid bronzers, cream bronzers are also extremely versatile!
- They can also be applied under or on top of foundation. They tend to be more pigmented than liquid bronzers so remember, a little goes a long way.
- Like cream blushes, they last quite long and act as a great base for powder bronzers.

 HOW TO APPLY: My preferred tool for applying cream bronzer is a medium sized, synthetic denser tapered kabuki brush.

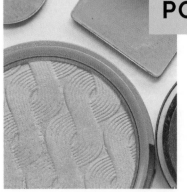

POWDERED BRONZER

- Powder bronzers are great to use when you don't have time to blend in a liquid or cream bronzer.
- Powder bronzers are one of my go-to beauty products because I come alive just a tad bit more than with just blush. I apply my bronzer under my cheekbones, up the corners of my face and beneath my jawline (think of a "3" pattern).
- I also use whatever bronzer is remaining on my brush to lightly shape my nose with the "W" pattern. Whatever is then left on the brush, I sweep onto my eyelids. Voila!

HOW TO APPLY: I normally use my natural hair blush brush to also apply bronzer. The angled medium face brush is another option.

BRONZER APPLICATION

APPLICATION 1 - THE DECOMPOSED "3"

During this bronzer application, think of the shapes of your "swoosh" like the parts of the number 3.

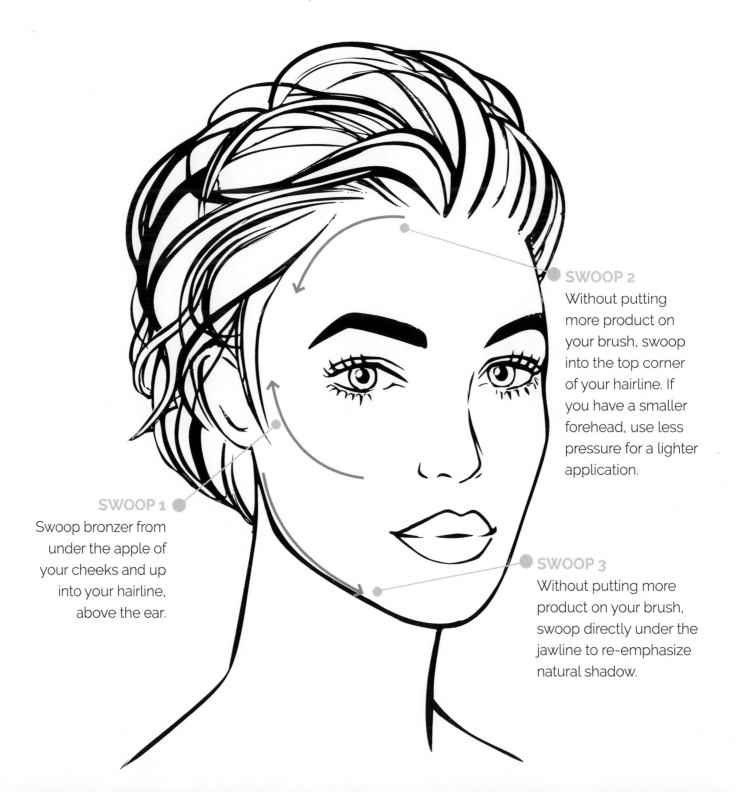

SWOOP 2
Without putting more product on your brush, swoop into the top corner of your hairline. If you have a smaller forehead, use less pressure for a lighter application.

SWOOP 1
Swoop bronzer from under the apple of your cheeks and up into your hairline, above the ear.

SWOOP 3
Without putting more product on your brush, swoop directly under the jawline to re-emphasize natural shadow.

BRONZER APPLICATION

APPLICATION 2 - THE DECOMPOSED "W"

On your second pass with bronzer, think of the shapes of your "swoosh" like the parts of the letter "w".

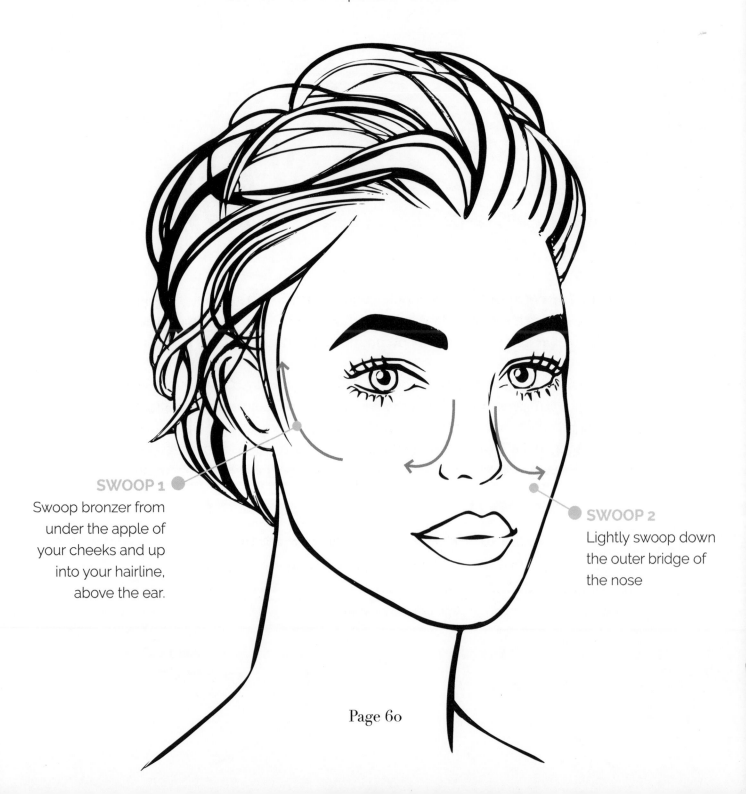

SWOOP 1
Swoop bronzer from under the apple of your cheeks and up into your hairline, above the ear.

SWOOP 2
Lightly swoop down the outer bridge of the nose

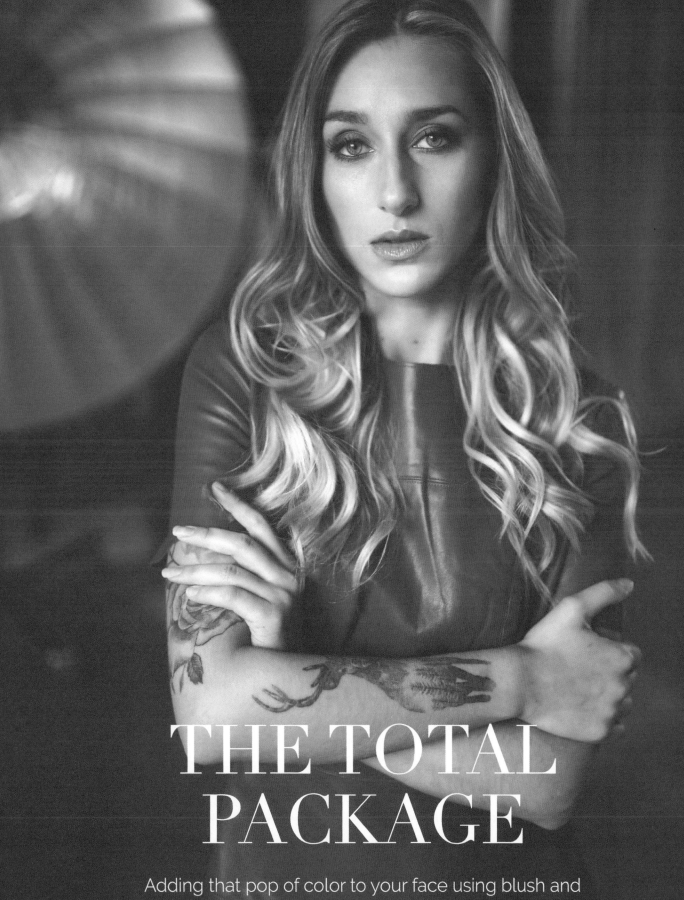

THE TOTAL PACKAGE

Adding that pop of color to your face using blush and bronzer is a great way to take your look to the next level. Remember, don't go overboard, keep it natural.

CONTOURING

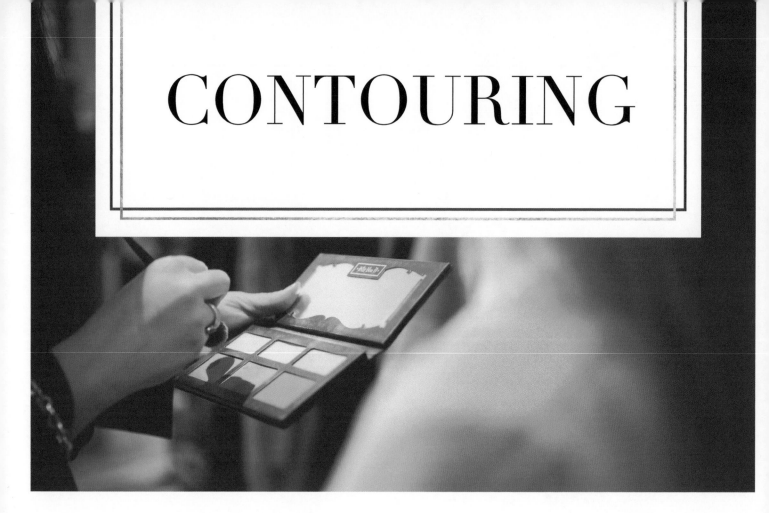

Contouring is also a popular and famous "stage makeup" technique that can alter the appearance of your face shape. Generally, contouring adds shadows to your face to give it the appearance of a slimmer, longer, and more accentuated shape.

Now, a little bit of "contouring" (aka face shaping) here and there is great for special occasions or some professional flash photography or even films, *but* day to day contouring is really something that is unnecessary and, when done improperly, looks disastrous. A good blush/bronzer/highlighter application negates the need for contouring, so focus your energies on that before diving into the world of contouring!

You do NOT need to buy a contour kit.
I repeat, you do NOT need to buy a contour kit!
(unless of course you are a professional makeup artist *or* love doing making on a wide range of skin tones).

CONTOUR APPLICATION

When "contouring" make sure to use a neutral shade a couple shades darker than your skin and always make sure to blend your contour extremely well into the ear and hairline.

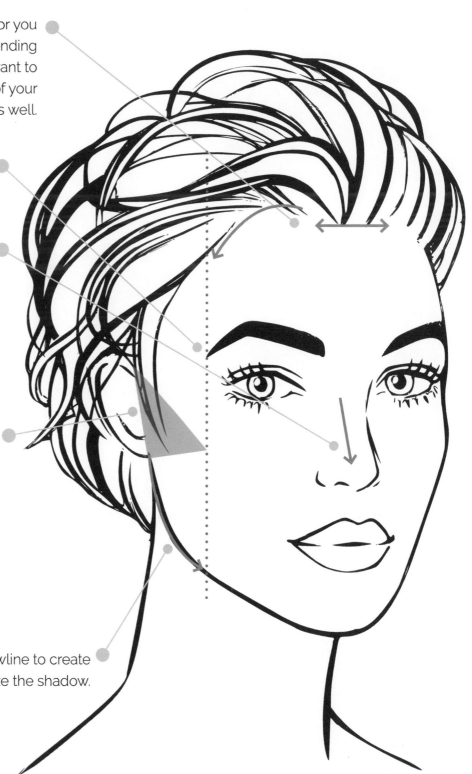

If you have a prominent forehead or you are wearing your hair up, depending on your face shape, you may want to consider "contouring:" the corners of your forehead and the length of it as well.

Never extend contour past the tip of your outer eyebrow.

You can also shape the nose to make it appear straighter, smaller, narrower. Parallel lines next to the bridge of the nose is a good place to start. Remember to blend, blend, blend should you choose to contour the nose.

When figuring out where to contour, make a peace sign with your fingers and place the middle finger where the top of your ear and face meet. Place your index finger where the end of your earlobe and face meet. This area may be visible to the naked eye if you have pronounced cheekbones.

Sweep the brush under the jawline to create and/or emphasize the shadow.

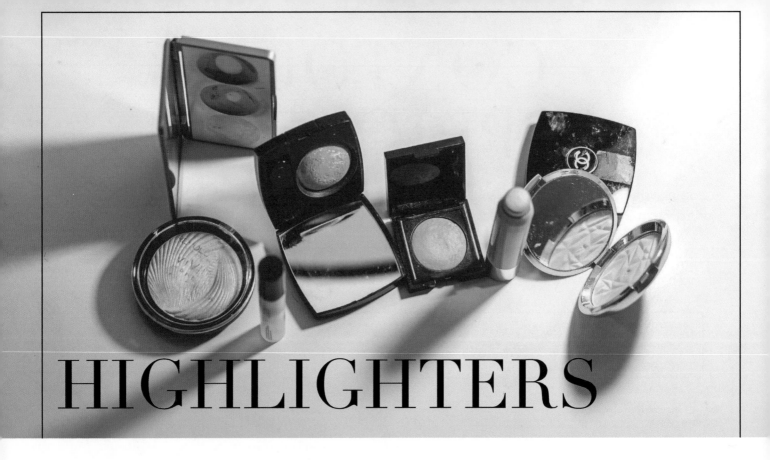

HIGHLIGHTERS

Blush adds the natural flush back to your face.

Bronzer adds sunkissed color back to your face.

Highlighters add that natural glow back to your face!

It's at this point in the makeup process where you really start to add the dimension back into your face and the magic really happens (and we haven't even gotten to the eyes yet!).

DOUBLE DUTY APPLICATION:

This product can pull double duty! *You can find blushes and bronzers that also act as highlighters (generally, they are baked and/or have metallic in them).*

This is great to save time getting ready but using a highlighter independent from blush and bronzer can create a polished and extremely put-together look!

*When you **practice practice practice**, you can get a good foundation, blush/bronzer/ highlight done in 2-3 minutes max. Don't feel discouraged, you've got this!*

NOT ALL HIGHLIGTHERS ARE CREATED EQUAL

WARM VS. COOL VS. NEUTRAL HIGHLIGHTER

This is where finding the right highlighter ties back into knowing your skin tone!

WARM TONES

COOL TONES

NEUTRAL TONES

If you are warm toned, you'll want to find highlighters that have more golden shimmer.

If you are cool toned, you'll want to find highlighters that have more silver shimmers.

If you are neutral toned, you'll want to find a highlighter that has more mixed metal.

Look for tones called:

Rose Gold

Sunrise/Sunset

Apricots/Peaches

Look for tones called:

Crushed Pearl

Moonlight/Starlight

Platinum

Look for tones called:

Opal

Champagne

Iridescent

LIQUID HIGHLIGHTER

- Less is always more with highlighter, especially liquid highlighter!
- You can dot on a few drops and press into skin until it's really blurred into the existing makeup.
- You can leave as-is for a natural, healthy glow or use that as a base for powder highlighter.

 HOW TO APPLY: It's best to apply liquid highlighter lightly from the fingertips in dots. Avoid "brushing" highlighter onto the face, as it is more difficult to blend, making the application process longer.

 TIP *Mix a touch of liquid highlighter into your foundation for a glowy, fresh look! If you have oily skin, keep in mind that this may appear more oily in photos.*

CREAM HIGHLIGHTER

- Used in somewhat the same way as liquid highlighters, cream highlighters are great for layering.
- Since creams are more pigmented, watch out.
- Applying a cream illuminator really adds a nice, healthy glow that lasts throughout the day!

 HOW TO APPLY: Like liquid highlighters, cream highlighters also can be worn under or on top of makeup and can be applied with the fingers, Applying cream highlighters on top of foundation may disturb the blush and/or bronzer,

POWDER HIGHLIGHTER

- Like a good cream blush or powder bronzer, a powder highlighter is one of my favorite makeup products. I can quickly and instantly add a beautiful and subtle glow to my face, even if I was out all day and I'm looking dull.
- **CAUTION:** Avoid highlighters with lots of glitter! Although they can look pretty upon application, by the end of the day, you may be left with a bunch of glitter and no sparkle.

 HOW TO APPLY: Apply your powdered highlighters with powder brush, a small domed (larger than eye smaller than face, not too dense) or a fan brush.

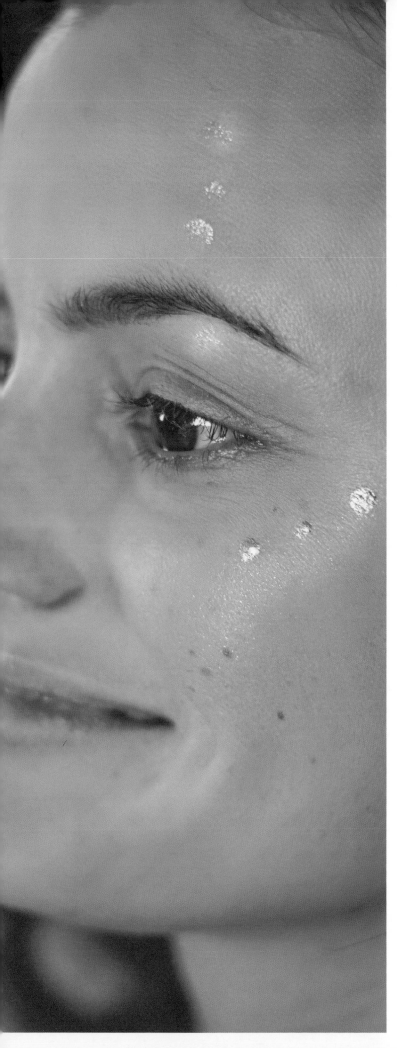

POPULAR HIGHLIGHTER APPLICATION TECHNIQUES

"UNDERPAINTING" HIGHLIGHTER OR "GLASS SKIN"

One thing I love to do is to "paint" the areas where light reflects (that I want to "highlight") before I apply foundation.

This allows a natural glow to peek through in areas extremely subtly. You can always intensify the effect by applying powder (or cream/liquid) highlighter on top.

This is also popularly known as "glass skin" which gives the appearance of such a natural finish to the skin, it shines like glass.

STROBING

Like contouring and baking, strobing is a technique that attempts to shape the face with strategic placement of only highlighters. Strobing is one of those "trends" that does take quite a bit of practice to look natural and flattering.

HIGHLIGHTER
APPLICATION

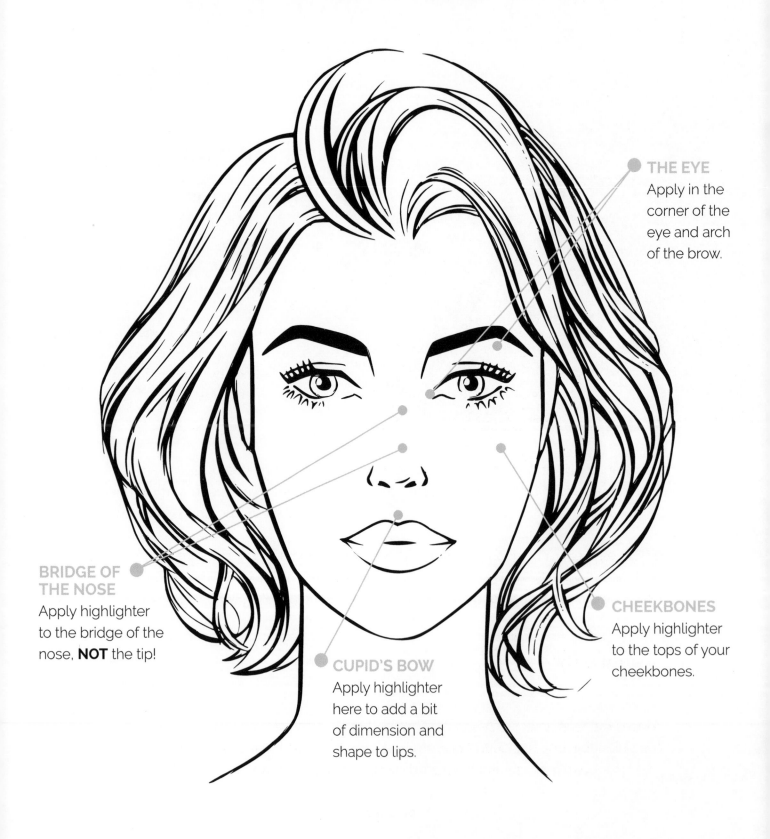

THE EYE
Apply in the corner of the eye and arch of the brow.

BRIDGE OF THE NOSE
Apply highlighter to the bridge of the nose, **NOT** the tip!

CUPID'S BOW
Apply highlighter here to add a bit of dimension and shape to lips.

CHEEKBONES
Apply highlighter to the tops of your cheekbones.

Beauty is not in the face; beauty is a light in the heart."

KAHLIL GIBRAN

EYE MAKEUP

THE READER'S DIGEST VERSION

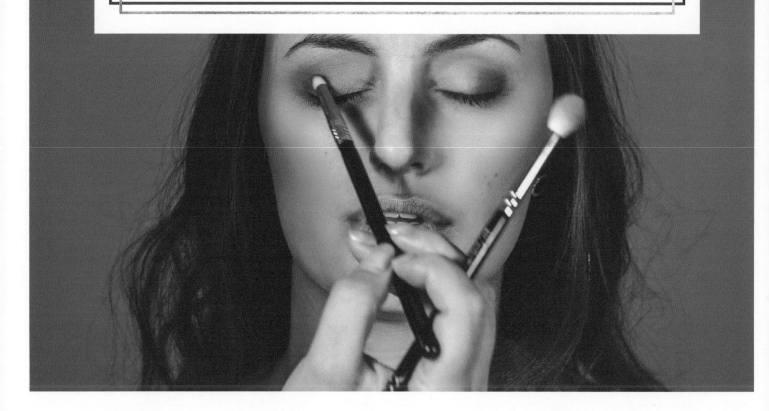

You may have golden undertones and cool, blue eyes or fair, cool pinkish undertones and warm amber honey eyes! Or you can be totally warm or totally cool -- which is absolutely gorgeous as well.

With face makeup, you learned about how and why you need to make sure all the colors compliment your skin tone. But when it comes to eye makeup, you might be able to pull off other colors around your eyes that don't necessarily fall into your skin tone color range.

This is why eyeshadow is SO much fun and also why you can break lots of the (non-existent) rules.

Entire books can be (and have been) written on eyeshadow, eyeliner, and eye shapes alone. This book covers the essentials for a daytime application and understanding eye makeup! It should give you a good springboard into the world of eye makeup!

TO THINE OWN EYE SHAPE BE TRUE...

Remember how knowing and loving your face shape is important? Knowing and respecting your eye shape is the most important aspect of eye makeup! This means that sometimes a simple eyeliner application, or a pop of color, or a little mascara can really be all that you need for day-to-day confidence! **Need inspiration?** Check out the celebrities under your eye shape to see how they make their eyes pop!

UPTURNED EYES
Kendall Jenner

Sophia Loren

  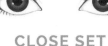

CLOSE SET EYES
Jennifer Anniston

Kristin Bell

MONOLID EYES
Lucy Liu

Maggie Q

DOWNTURNED EYES
Anne Hathaway

Katie Holmes

WIDE SET EYES
Oprah

Rihanna

  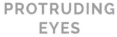

PROTRUDING EYES
Nicole Richie

Mila Kunis

ROUND EYES
Katy Perry

Natalie Setareh

   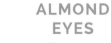

ALMOND EYES
Beyonce

Ariana Grande (also close set)

HOODED EYES
Taylor Swift

Jennifer Lawrence

PRIMER & SHADOW

Just like you prep and create a beautiful base for makeup application on the face, you will want to create a beautiful base on the eyes. Many of the same rules still apply and you'll be shocked to learn exactly how easy eye makeup can be on the daily with the important information found in this section!

THE TWO STEP EYE MAKEUP PROCESS

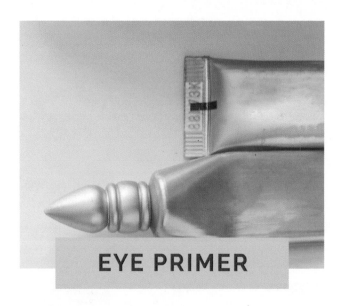

EYE PRIMER

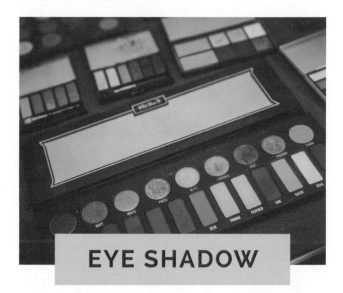

EYE SHADOW

Like face primers, eye primers are not a necessity, but are great to have on-hand for more dramatic eye looks or eye makeup you need to last all day. **For Normal or Dry Eyelids:** a liquid concealer may be a great substitute for primer in evening out the skin tone of the eye and prepping it for eyeshadow application. **For Oily Eyelids:** you'll need to use an eye primer almost anytime you plan on wearing eye makeup, as the eye makeup will likely crease or melt off. Look for eye primers (or regular primers) that are mattifying and oil free.

The most important rule in eyeshadow application is that there are no rules! The sky is the limit, and knowing your eye's complimentary colors (warm vs. cool) will help narrow your selection in a palette heavy industry. Keep in mind that you may have warm undertones but blue eyes with cool undertones. Invest in building a good matte palette and a good metallic palette. That should last you for years! On the following pages, you'll learn all about what colors work for you and also, which types of eyeshadow formulas are ideal for your eye shape and skin type!

EXPERT
SHADOW GUIDE

Did you know that there's an ideal shadow shade for your eye color?
Complimentary colors are 1-2 shades darker or lighter than your eye color.
A great "pop" of color is a color opposite your eye color on the color wheel!
Now, grab your color wheel, find your eye color and have some fun exploring!

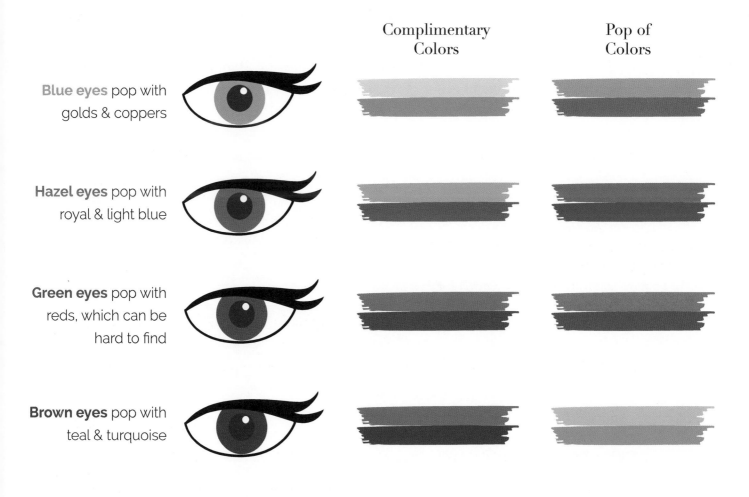

	Complimentary Colors	Pop of Colors
Blue eyes pop with golds & coppers		
Hazel eyes pop with royal & light blue		
Green eyes pop with reds, which can be hard to find		
Brown eyes pop with teal & turquoise		

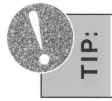

TIP: ***Buyer beware!*** *Most eyeshadow palettes are designed to appeal to lots of different people with lots of different skin tones! Be extremely discerning when purchasing eyeshadow palettes -- as most of the colors may not work for you!*

Page 73

SHADOW FINISHES

Like all the other products we've discussed in this book, eyeshadows come in quite a few different formulas! The most popular formulas are powders, creams, crayons, and loose pigments. They also have a variety of finishes, including Matte, Metallic, Frost, Shimmer, Satin, Lustre, Marble, Metallic.

GENERAL RULE OF THUMB

As we age, we should avoid the glitters and shimmers, as they can collect in fine lines and wrinkles! Although if glitter is your thing, SHINE ON at any age! Make sure you are using a quality eye glitter cosmetic grade adhesive, okay?

When purchasing eyeshadows or palettes, make sure you have a balance of shadow types, colors, and textures that are flattering on **YOU!**

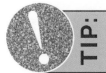 **TIP:** *Buying makeup pans, as opposed to pre-made palettes saves you quite a bit of money — that is of course, if you are okay without all the packaging!*

 **RESOURCE** *Make your own palettes by depotting your favorite shadows and putting them in a magnetic palette. **Z-palettes** are one of the most popular magnetized palettes and come in a variety of shapes and sizes. Once you create your signature look, you can put everything you need in one palette (blush, bronzer, highlighter, and shadows). You can find lots of tutorial videos on how-to depot your makeup and there are even depotting kits available.*

ALL GLITTER LESS PIGMENT

GLITTER

LUSTER

SHIMMER

FROST

| MATTE | SATIN | METALLIC | FROST |

NO GLITTER NO SPARKLE NO SHINE

NO GLITTER LOTS OF SPARKLE & SHINE

EYE SHADOW APPLICATION

For eyes and depending on your preferences, you'll need blending brushes of all sizes. Remember, using a cream shadow underneath will help the eyeshadow pop and also make it last longer.

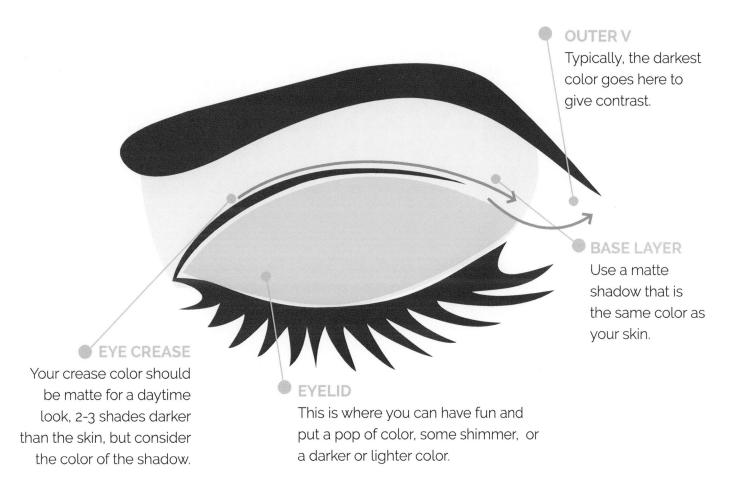

OUTER V
Typically, the darkest color goes here to give contrast.

BASE LAYER
Use a matte shadow that is the same color as your skin.

EYE CREASE
Your crease color should be matte for a daytime look, 2-3 shades darker than the skin, but consider the color of the shadow.

EYELID
This is where you can have fun and put a pop of color, some shimmer, or a darker or lighter color.

HAVE CLOSE SET EYES?
Think of light to dark moving from the inner corner to the outer corners (top and bottom).

HAVE HOODED EYES?
Matte shadows are your friend. Concentrate eyeshadow directly above the pupil and blend horizontally across the eye and outwards.

HAVE ALMOND EYES?
These eyes are proportionate and the sky is the limit in playing with techniques.

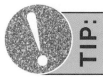 **TIP:** ***The number one rule of eye shadow application is "don't forget to blend" and blend lots!*** *Blending makes smoother transitions and creates a beautiful finished look.*

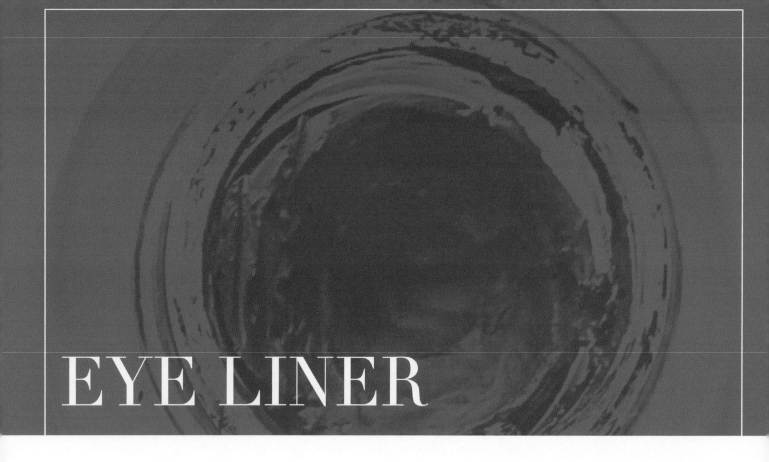

EYE LINER

Aside from concealer, eyeliner is probably one of the most used and abused items in makeup. Precise eye line application that suits your eye shape (and personality) requires a steady hand, lots of practice, and wait, did I mention lots of practice?

Don't be deceived by everything you see on the Internet -- eyeliner is something that, if applied improperly, can age you 10-15 years or can make your eyes appear small and beady.

READY TO DIG IN, AND PERHAPS, UNLEARN EVERYTHING YOU THOUGHT YOU KNEW ABOUT EYELINER?

TIP

Traditional eyeliners (black, gray, brown, plum, navy) help to make the white of your eyes appear whiter and your lashes longer. Eyeliner creates a sort of color block, which is why, when eyeliner is applied correctly, it can appear as if your eye shape changes!

WHAT TYPE OF EYELINER SHOULD I USE?

Eye lining was originally invented to make the eyelashes appear longer and eyes bigger. Eyeliner is often applied AFTER eye shadow to complete and tie in the entire eye look, but again, there are no rules!

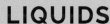

LIQUIDS

Liquid eyeliner is probably the hardest eyeliner to master. Applying liquid liner requires the most steady hand and lots of practice, that is if you want your liner to look amazing and semi-symmetric. You can also turn your powder and gels into liquids with special thinners and apply with a fine tipped brush, a great way to maximize your existing stash. Don't share your liquid liner with anyone! Also, liquids can be quite unflattering on those who have thin skin or lots of wrinkles around the eyes.

GELS

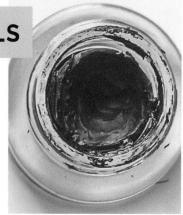

Similar to liquids, gels require skill and practice, but gels are a bit more flexible in the application. Adele's signature eyeliner is done with a gel liner! Gels require a precision (generally synthetic) brush to apply. Can be "set" with a powder to soften and/or intensify. This is *my* preferred eyeliner application for evening events.

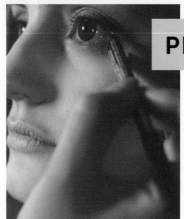

PENCILS

The most versatile and convenient eyeliner application! Eyeliner pencil technology has come a long way and now, you can get long-lasting, waterproof pencil eyeliners. Although you won't get the precise tip that you could get with liquids and gels, you and get pretty deep into the lash line, night light (if you want), and even use pencils to create a smoky eye in a pinch! Works on all ages!

POWDERS

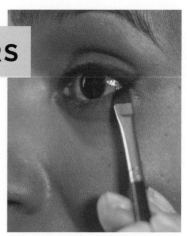

You will need a small angled eyeliner brush in order to apply powder eyeliner. This does require a bit of practice but the mistakes aren't as hard to correct compared to using gels or liquids. Lining your eyes with a powder liner creates the softest, most natural eyeline of the bunch! This option is also great for "setting" your liquid or gel.

PRO EYELINER HACKS

START THIN: Applying a thin layer of eyeliner starting deep into the lash line (and even the tightline) will instantly open your eyes, regardless of eye shape. You can always build it and go more bold for a dramatic evening look.

CURL THOSE LASHES: Eyelash curlers are probably the best tool for instantly opening up the eyes and it requires zero makeup! If you don't have time for mascara or eyeshadow, a quick eyelash curl can do wonders!

OPEN THOSE EYES: A lot of women make the mistake of applying gorgeous eye makeup when their eyes are closed, and when they open them, it looks like a hot mess. It's important to apply your eye makeup, especially eyeliner, looking straight forward into the mirror **IN ADDITION TO** applying on a semi-closed eye. You can gently pull the skin of the eye outward to eliminate the wrinkles, but remember to be gentle here and fill in the eyeliner with the skin relaxed to guarantee a smooth line.

EYELINER
APPLICATION GUIDE

LASHLINE
Should be the same color as tightline if tightline is visible with eyes open.

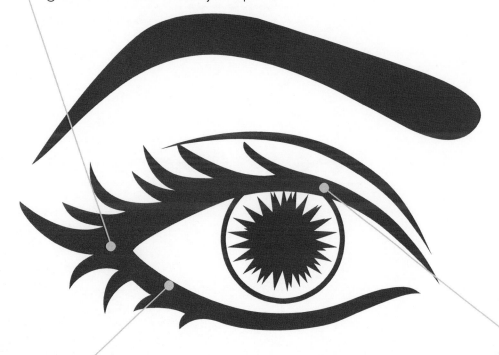

TIGHTLINE
line dark to make eyes appear larger and eyelashes longer. Sometimes simply lining the tightline is enough, especially for big eyes or monolid eyes. It's important to keep your eyeliner pencil (best for lining tightline) extremely clean and sanitized.

WATERLINE
Line dark for a sexy/moody look or line light for a brighter look.

EYELINER
STYLE GUIDE

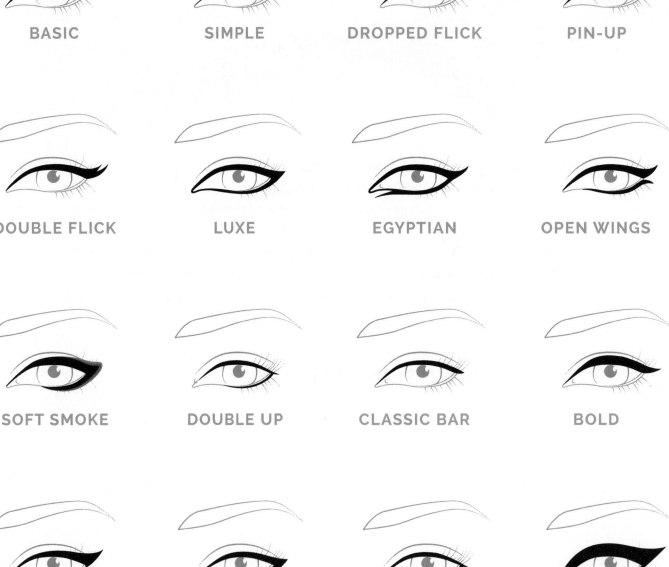

BASIC

SIMPLE

DROPPED FLICK

PIN-UP

DOUBLE FLICK

LUXE

EGYPTIAN

OPEN WINGS

SOFT SMOKE

DOUBLE UP

CLASSIC BAR

BOLD

FELINE

ARABIC

SLEPT-IN SMUDGE

ARABIC

LASHES
FOR DAYS

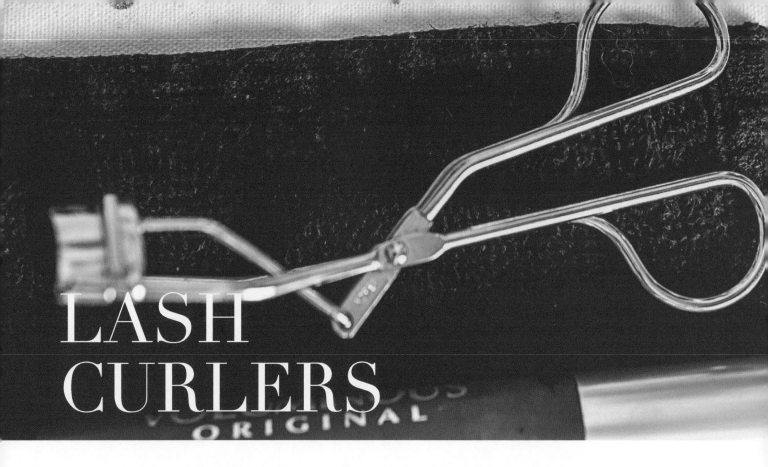

LASH CURLERS

While the eyelash curler may look and seem like a torture device, fear not. The only way to really hurt yourself is to curl your eyelashes in a moving car (don't do it) or curl your eyelashes while watching a scary movie.

There are so many different types of eyelash curlers on the market! The one pictured here is a traditional, full-sized eyelash curler. However, you can also use half-sized eyelash curlers, mini eyelash curlers, and even heated ones.

TIPS FOR CURLING LASHES

PINCH NOT: *The closer to the lash bed, the more risk of "pinching" however, because YOU control the pressure, you'd feel if you were too close. If it feels too close, move outward from the lash bed.*

FIND YOUR SWEET SPOT: *I like to curl lashes right in the middle of the lash, far enough away from the lash bed that I'm not scared of pinching myself but also far enough from the edge to actually get a noticeable curl.*

NOT ALL LASH CURLERS ARE CREATED EQUAL: *I used a curler for years, having to squeeze and hold 3-4 times per side. I thought that was normal... until I upgraded my eyelash curler and realized I could achieve a perfect curl in 1-2 clamps per side.*

MASCARA CLAIMS

Mascara is the one makeup item that I feel naked without. It creates that visual separation between the eye and the whites of the eye faster than eyeliner. Mascara makes the eyes pop with a few sweeps of pigments and mascara is hands down one of the most affordable and accessible makeup products for anyone!!

The thing is... the actual formulas of mascaras are pretty much the same, unless of course you need a waterproof or tubing mascara. When shopping for mascara, remember it's the brush you are buying!

There's an abundance of information on the internet but we often tend to buy mascara blindly based on packaging and/or claims! It's important to know which types of brushes to expect with different types of claims.

CLAIM	IDEAL LASH TYPE	IDEAL BRUSH	RESULT
CURL	Straight, thin lashes or thicker lashes that already have a slight curl but need a little more!	Curved Brush	May or may not live up to the claims, especially depending on your eyelash type. Eyelash curlers are best bet. Chunkier lash is to be expected.
LENGTHEN	Light colored, thin or thick lashes that simply need length.	Narrow Brush Pinecone Brush	These mascaras will make your lashes look more wispy and separated. It helps the lashes appear longer, but not necessarily thicker. This is a great option for lower lashes!
THICKEN	Great for long, thin lashes!	Chunky/Thick Brush	Thickening mascaras make lashes LOOK thicker because the brush creates a chunkier application.
VOLUMIZING	All lashes can benefit with this type of formula but not necessarily "excel" in one area.	Medium, Straight Brush	The result can be chunkier lashes, if that's your thing. Otherwise you might want to comb out the lashes post-application.

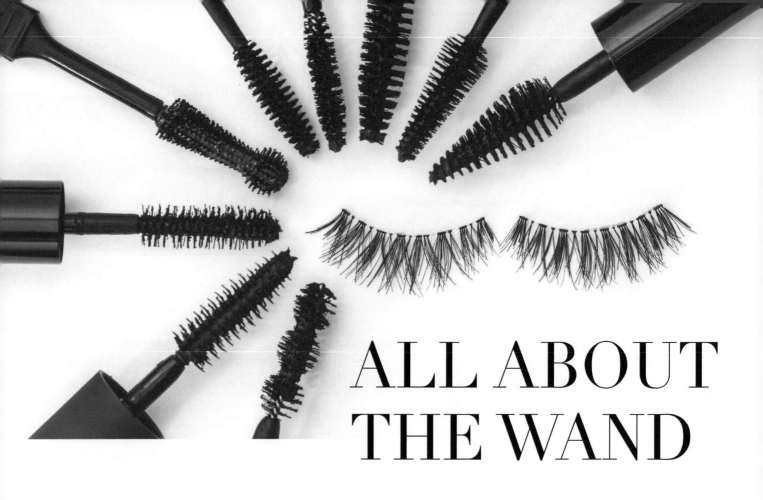

ALL ABOUT THE WAND

There are LOTS of different brushes out there. These are the most common and widely available brushes (but not all inclusive). The thicker the wand and brush, the easier it is to "mess up." When you mess up on your mascara, **DON'T PANIC.** I'll share tips on what to do on the next page!

OVERSIZED THICK WAND	PINE CONE WAND	CURVED WAND	FLAT COMB WAND	MICRO WAND	RUBBER SHORTY	BALL TIPPED
Creates max. volume	*Cat eye corners*	*Curls Lashes*	*Separated & Dark*	*Tinted but Natural*	*Define Length*	*Detailed Corners*

"MESS UP" YOUR MASCARA?

REMEMBER! Don't panic. Don't immediately try to rub it off. Just breathe, move onto the next eye OR your lips. Wait for it to dry, then follow these tips to fix it!

REMOVING NON-WATERPROOF MASCARA

Most non-waterproof mascaras will flake off extremely easily with the tip of a cotton swab. You can do this without disturbing makeup and then easily reapply. This is advice I learned way too late in life!

REMOVING WATERPROOF MASCARA

If the trick above doesn't work, try applying a bit of your moisturizer cream, letting it set for 30 seconds and lightly rubbing it off. You may need to use your foundation brush or eye blending brush to re-blend everything in -- but with some patience and grace, you'll make the "mistake" disappear!

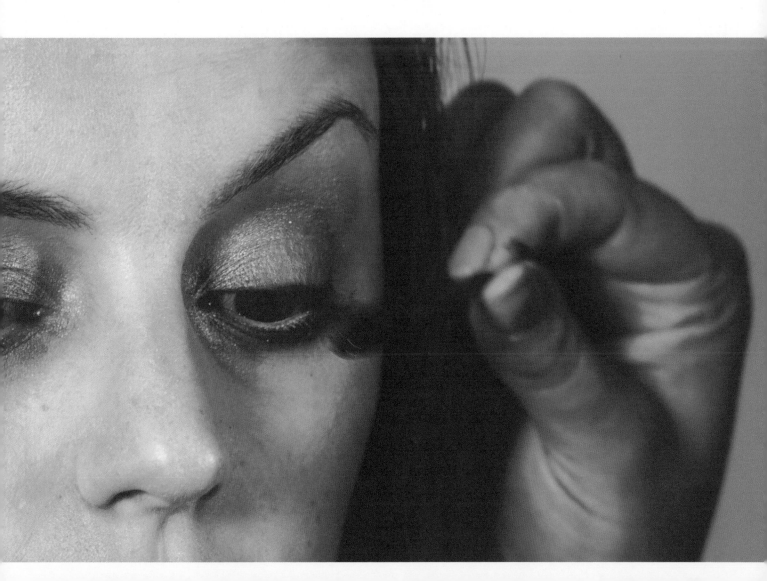

MASCARA TYPES

DISCLAIMER: When you're buying mascara, check out the ingredient list. As with any product, all mascaras are not created equal. You'll definitely want to look and see where "water" falls into the ingredient list (you might have to contact the mascara manufacturer directly to get that information). If water is one of the first few ingredients, it will probably run. If water is one of the last ingredients, it will probably flake off. Find a mascara where water is in a happy place!

CURLING MASCARA

Curling mascaras help to curl the lashes. They typically come with a curved brush. These types of mascaras have a pretty standard application and your lashes won't be too thick or too long. Don't 100% rely on your mascara to curl your lash. Instead curl your eyelashes with a proper eyelash curler and find a mascara that further accentuates your curled lashes.

TUBING MASCARA

A tubing mascara will coat each lash with water resistant mascara, great for sensitive/teary eyes, humid climates and short/fine/downward pointing lashes. If you apply more than one coat, it will likely be extremely clumpy!

Once you find the type of brush and formula you like the best, it'll make shopping for mascara much less intimidating and you'll know exactly which brush and "claim" to look for specifically for your eye shape, lash type, and of course personal preferences!

TIPS

Eco Friendly / Alternate Application: You can buy a cream mascara and apply it with an actual brush! Use a mini fan brush. This allows you to get super close to the lash line and comb out. Great for up-close (aka macro) beauty shots!

Clumps got your down?: You can comb out lashes with a lash comb or a clean mascara spoolie. Don't have a spoolie? Clean and cut off an old mascara wand and make your own. It's better for the environment too!

RESOURCE

Besame is a company that specializes in recreating vintage makeup classics. They sell cream mascara and a reusable mascara wand. Not only is this better for the environment but it looks super chic and hipster, if that's your thing!

MASCARA APPLICATION

The outer lashes are what really open up your eyes! It's important to focus on these lashes. Use the tip of the wand to find the outermost corner and then angle the wand back (flipping it 180 degrees) to really get deep into the lash bed and fan the lashes out and up.

Hold the brush parallel to the eyelashes at the center of the eye, getting as close to the lash bed as possible and winging out and up!

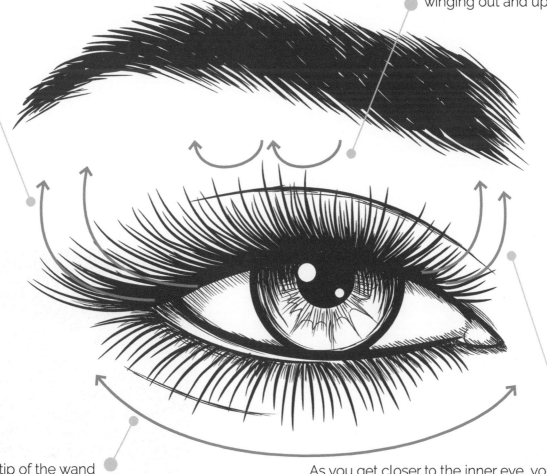

Use the tip of the wand to brush lightly over the bottom lashes from edge to edge.

As you get closer to the inner eye, you'll need to angle the wand to remain parallel, using the tip of the wand to get the tiny, oftentimes lighter lashes.

FALSE LASHES

TYPES & APPLICATIONS

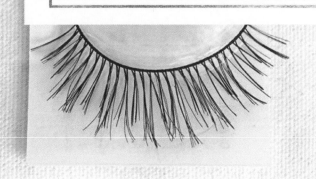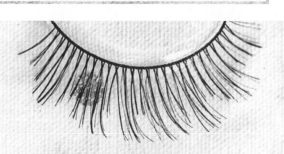

False lashes have grown in popularity in recent years. They are such a fun option for anyone who has the time, energy, and patience to learn how to apply them. There are so many different types of false lashes, and a new type emerges seemingly daily.

COMMON MATERIALS	LASH "SIZES"	PROPER CARE
Human Hair	Full Strip	Real Hair Lashes, with proper care, are reusable, up to a specified time frame.
Animal Hair	Half Strip	
(commonly mink or silk)	Individual Lashes	
Plastic/Synthetic		Plastic/Synthetic lashes are designed for one time use.

My Advice: If you love how you look in false lashes, invest in a pair of reusable ones you like -- it's better for the environment, there's less packaging waste, and you'll get a nice "broken in" natural lash look.

If you have a one-off special occasion and feel like your mascara (primer + three solid coats of fiber mascara) isn't doing the trick, try a synthetic lash. or just applying single lashes to the outer corners or in between sparse lashes.

LASH APPLICATION

If you don't have time to apply your falsies correctly, **DON'T DO IT!** Not only is it unflattering, improper application can result in lashes falling off, lashes scratching the eye, bacteria collecting in places it shouldn't. So here's the step by step for strip lashes (since they are the most popular). Don't skip steps UNLESS you have already well-fitted lashes.

1. Curl your natural lashes to match the curl of the falsies as much as possible.
2. Apply mascara to your natural lashes before applying your falsies. Do NOT apply mascara to your falsies if you want to use your falsies more than once.
3. **SIZE YOUR LASHES!** If you buy strip lashes, they need to be sized to YOUR eye. Period. Unless your natural eyeline is visibly longer than the strip, you must size the lashes to your eyes before application.
   Size by placing the inner corner of the falsie to the inner corner of your eyeline. Find where your natural eyeline stops and mark where you need to trim the end of the falsie.
4. Apply a thin coat of lash glue to the falsie and wait 30 seconds or so for it to get tacky.
5. Hover the lash over the center of the eye and find perfect placement
6. LOOK DOWN to apply your eyelash. Don't apply false eyelashes with your eyes closed (for obvious reasons #glue).
7. Adjust the falsie as close to the lash bed as possible in the next 30 seconds (before the glue dries). THIS IS EXTREMELY IMPORTANT if you want the falsie to look seamless.
8. Finally, you **must** apply a thin coat of eyeliner on top for a polished finish.

WHAT ABOUT LASH EXTENSIONS?

Like with anything, doing your research is important if you're considering eyelash extensions! You also get what you pay for! Find a reputable esthetician who has loads of experience, follows sanitation and hygiene, and has great referrals.

I think eyelash extensions are great for brides who have a jam-packed wedding weekend plus honeymoon post-wedding. Why? They don't have to worry about mascara, at all! They can cry all they want, jump into pool, kiss under waterfalls, or play in the rain -- and not have to worry about their mascara running, chunking up, or even applying it at all.

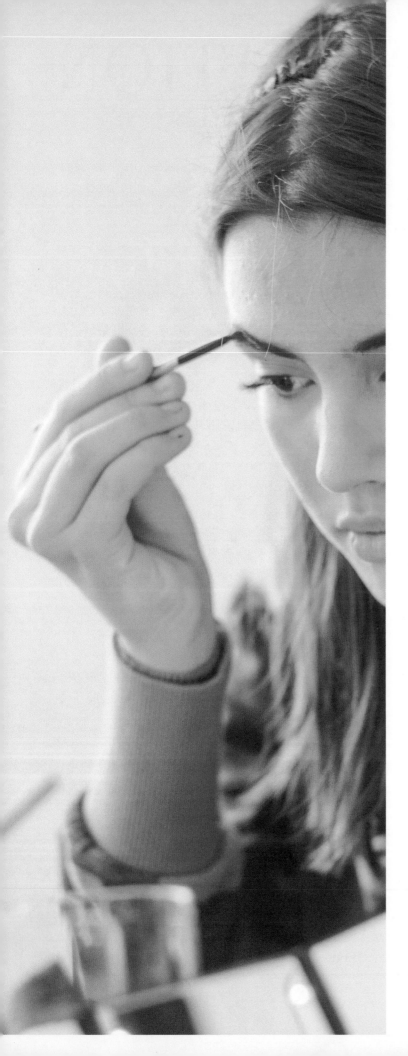

BROWS

Everyone says that eyes are the window to the soul but really, your eyebrows frame your eyes and are therefore the foundation to the eyes, the face, and well -- they are basically really important. Some makeup artists start with brows first, because they are so important in understanding the face shape. To each their own, all brows deserve attention, some more than others.

If you grew up in the 90s or even early 2000s and you kept up with trends, you likely over plucked your eyebrows! Sadly, eyebrow hairs are hard to grow back or fill in!

My philosophy on brows, especially if you are victim to the thin eyebrow trend, is to lay off the tweezers. Sure you can pluck those wild hairs that are obviously way out of the lane but patience is a virtue.

QUICK & PAINLESS EYEBROWS

Combing & grooming the brows is just as important as filling them in! A clear mascara wand or clear eyebrow brush works wonders, especially if you applied foundation. You don't have to spend a lot of money on fancy eyebrow products, unless of course you are an eyebrow girl or guy.

A NOTE ON MICROBLADING

For those of you whose brows are not super defined or visible, microblading may be an investment worth saving for. Microblading is a semi-permanent tattoo that, if done well by a trusted professional, will save you lots of time, money, and energy in the long run! **Remember** again, "you get what you pay for."

BROW FORMULAS

Just like eyeliners, there's different types of brow products. The key to brows is blending and making them look natural. This again, takes practice and patience and more practice. Knowing your face and eye shape will help in determining what brow shape suits you!

For any/every brow product, I recommend using a coarse angled brush (synthetic for creams and blending liquids or natural hair brushes for the powders) AND a spoolie. **The spoolie is essential to making sure the brow makeup is blended well.**

PAINTS & LIQUIDS

Brow paints & liquid eyebrow liners are products I generally steer clear of. When applied improperly, the eyebrows rarely look natural. Unless you need a specific look for a theatrical performance or an editorial shoot, avoid these.

GELS

I love eyebrow gels that come in mascara tubes. They make for an easy application and blend nicely.

Apply with an angled synthetic brow brush.

PENCILS

Liquid and dry pencils are great to draw hairs in sparse areas. Avoid pressing down hard and swiping left and right; draw individual brow hairs in an upward motion, matching the angle of your existing brow hairs! Don't forget to spoolie in between sets.

POWDERS

Powder eyeliners are buildable, look natural, and best of all, are easy to remove!

Apply with coarse small angled eye brush. "Swipe" along the bottom and top of the brow and blend in until smooth; for a good match, you may need to blend 2-3 shades.

TIPS

***ALWAYS** match your brows to your natural hair color. Sometimes you might have to mix colors to get a perfect match, and that's okay.*
***If you have oily skin,** make sure to prime the eyebrows with an oil-free primer and "set" the brows with a clear brow gel*
***Double Duty:** Matte eye shadows can double as eyebrow powders!*

BROW SHAPE GUIDE

Did you know you had an eyebrow shape too? Here are a few suggestions if you're struggling to find the right look for your brows! Match these brow shapes with your face shape, which you should have identified earlier in this book.

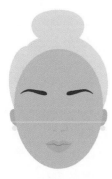

Soft and angled brows are best for those with an **oval shaped face**.

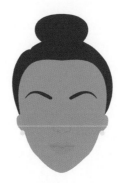

If you have a **triangle shaped face**, try thin and rounded brows with longer tails.

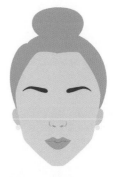

Soften a **diamond shaped face** with curved eyebrows. This lessens the width of the widest part of the face.

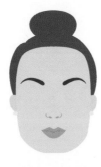

For those with a **rectangle shaped face**, thicker brows and softer arches help to soften the face shape.

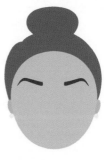

If you have a **round shaped faced**, high arches will draw the eye upward to make the face appear longer.

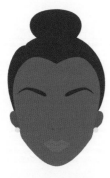

Have a **heart shaped face**? Try a low arch with round and curved brows

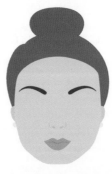

For a **square shaped face**, the stronger the angles of the face, the stronger the curve of the brow should be.

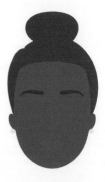

If you have an **oblong shaped face,** flatter eyebrows will make the face appear shorter

HOW TO SHAPE YOUR BROWS

There is no "one size fits all" brow formula to follow, but the diagram pictured below outlines the general proportions you should follow. Ultimately, you want your brow shape, which you just identified on the last page, to compliment your face shape.

TRY THIS THREE PART BROW-SHAPING METHOD

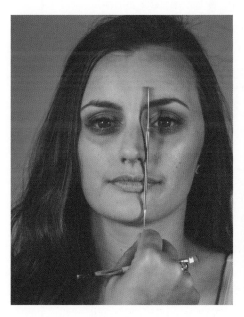 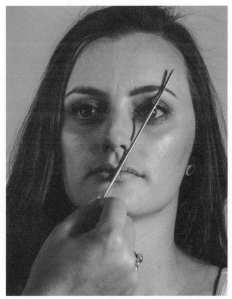 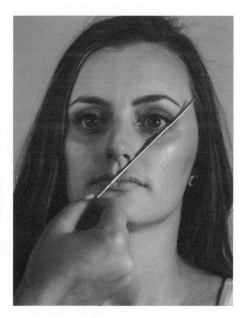

LINE A

To find where the inside edge of your brow should fall, create a vertical line from the edge of the nose. Your brow should reach this line, but not go past it.

LINE B

To locate where the center of your natural arch should fall, create a straight line at a 45 degree angle from the edge of the nose through the center of the eye.

LINE C

For the outer edge of your brow, create a diagonal line from the edge of the nose to the edge of your eye. Your brow should reach this line, but not go past it.

"Eyebrows... the one thing you can get into shape without exercising."

UNKNOWN

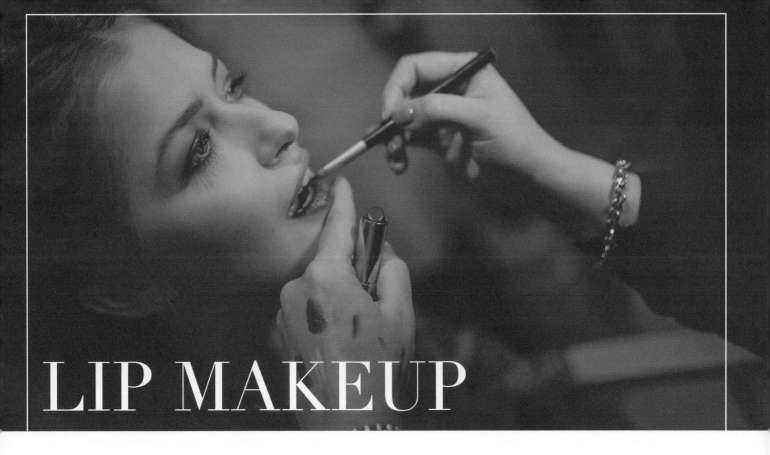

LIP MAKEUP

More than eye shadow, changing your lip color is probably the easiest way to change your entire look in a pinch! We tend to notice people who wear bold lipsticks, for better or for worse! Adding a bold lipstick to any look automatically changes the tone of your look.

As we get older, our lip color dulls and they tend to "shrink." That's probably why we remember our grandmothers distinctive lip colors they wore down to the core.

BOLD LIPS, BOLD EYES, OR BOTH?

Remember what I said? There are no hard rules when it comes to makeup, makeup is an art. It's *your* form of self-expression! So if you want to go bold and make a statement, go for it! However, I like to think of Coco Chanel's famous quote

"Before you leave the house, look in the mirror and take one thing off."

This can be an accessory, that extra bit of blush, those extra bobby pins, that bracelet or necklace, even those eyelashes!

Personally, finding balance between your eye makeup and lipstick is the most popular and comfortable way I prefer to keep balance in any makeup look I do.

For example, if you have a heavy eye, try going with a lighter lip closest to your natural lip color or maybe a bit on the nude side. If you are wanting a bold lip, then maybe keep your eye makeup simple. A good coat of mascara can generally do the trick!

FIND YOUR SHADE

Choosing the right shades of red and pink can be tough and wearing a new color can be uncomfortable in general. If you want to ease into a new shade, try mixing or lightening the shade you want to wear with a shade that you already wear. That way you'll ease into the new color and eventually be able to rock whatever color. You too can rock a bold lip with baby steps.

A quick note about nude shades! Nudes can be the best and worst shades. So many women just skip their lipstick and apply lip-gloss or chapstick over their lips that have been covered with foundation and/or powder. Though this may work when you are a teenager, it doesn't necessarily mean it will work as you age, or if you want to look alive in photos.

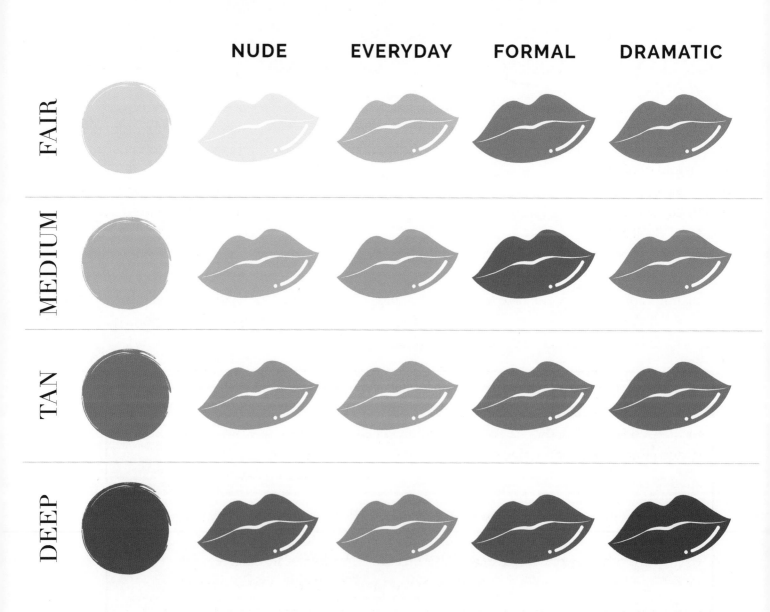

TYPES OF LIPSTICK

NO SHINE TO HIGH SHINE

These types of lipstick can be found in every shade under the sun. Here are a few notes to help you find the best type for you and your skin.

TYPE	FINISH	APPLICATION NOTES
PAINTS & LONG LASTING	Generally matte; no shine	Wear chapstick under or add on top to add moisture and dimension; add gloss for shine and extra moisture.
MATTE	No shine	Can dry out lips, good to mix with chapstick for added moisture; not as long lasting as a paint but also not as damaging; goes on quite a bit dryer.
CREAM	Natural shine	Great versatile lipstick right in the middle; just enough natural shine and balance in the formula; not super long lasting but also not going to rub off super easily; mostly made with vegetable wax!
SATIN/SHEER	Not as shiny or sparkly as pearls/ frosted lipsticks	Not long-lasting; goes on quite slick; lots more oil in these lipsticks.
PEARL/ FROSTED	Sparkle and shine all day long!	Sometimes can leave your lips dry; wear or mix pearls/ frosted lipsticks with mattes to make your own new custom lipstick!
GLOSS	High shine	A gloss is a great way to make smaller lips appear larger! Apply glosses on nude lips or on top of lipstick for added pop and dimension!

TIP

*Lip Care 101: Chapsticks are essentially moisturizer for your lips! Protect the delicate skin of your lips by applying as needed or before lipstick application (can help lipstick glide on easier, but may also compromise longevity of lip color). Especially important if you live in drier climates or during the dry seasons (summers and winters). **Don't forget SPF on those lips either.***

LIPSTICK APPLICATION

DEFYING GRAVITY!

Most of us are used to applying lipstick on our upper lip in a downward motion. The "streak" and the flow of the lipstick then faces downwards. I encourage you to flip this and paint 'up.'

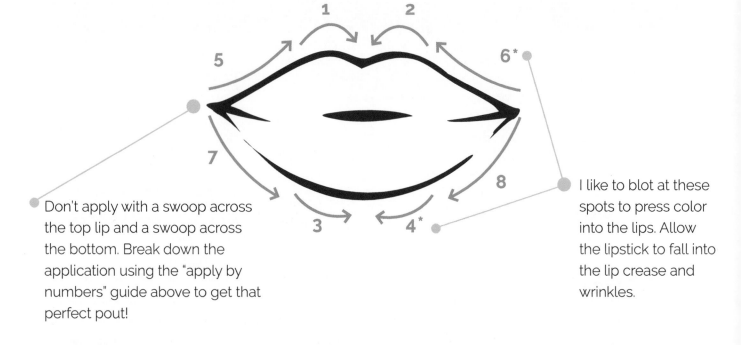

Don't apply with a swoop across the top lip and a swoop across the bottom. Break down the application using the "apply by numbers" guide above to get that perfect pout!

I like to blot at these spots to press color into the lips. Allow the lipstick to fall into the lip crease and wrinkles.

TIPS

Got lipstick on your teeth? Vaseline can be used on the teeth to keep your lipstick from transferring onto your teeth but you can also just lightly put your pointer finger into your mouth and lightly pull out (sounds so dirty!). If Vaseline isn't your thing, try coconut oil. Just brush a light coat onto your front 4 teeth with your lip brush or dab on with your finger tips.

Blotting is KEY! It is SO important that you remember to blot your lips after applying lipstick. Not only does blotting help to stain your lips and keep that lip color in place, it also fills in all the tiny little nooks and crannies of the lips. So you can apply, blot, reapply, blot, apply, blot & bam!

LIP LINERS

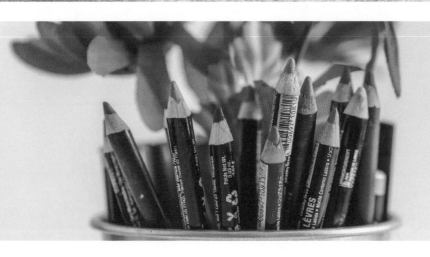

Technically you'd line your lips before applying lipstick but that's only if you wear lip liner! You might not need it or might not have the time.

Lining your lips can really amplify your lip makeup game! Not only does lining your lips (especially if you fill them in) help your lip color to last longer, it really makes for a more complete lip look and you can "change" the shape of your lip without fillers, botox, or surgery.

Don't worry, you don't need to rush out and find exact color matches for all your favorite lipsticks. You can get a generic red, generic pink, a generic nude, and a generic plum or coral (just the shade families that you like to wear, more or less) and that will generally match a similar shade in lipstick. Liners tend to blend easily, which is an important step not to forget!

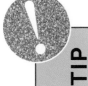

TIP

A lip liner is NOT necessary when applying lip paints. Lip paints are extremely matte, opaque, and last an extremely long time -- therefore rendering lip liners redundant!

LINING FOR YOUR LIP SHAPE

We already learned that as we age, we lose skin elasticity, and our lips are no exception.

Lip liner is that perfect solution for lips that have lost some of their fullness and shape over time!

Not only that, but lip liner can also give you an instant lip lift with proper application, which is always fun for those days you want to feel fancy.

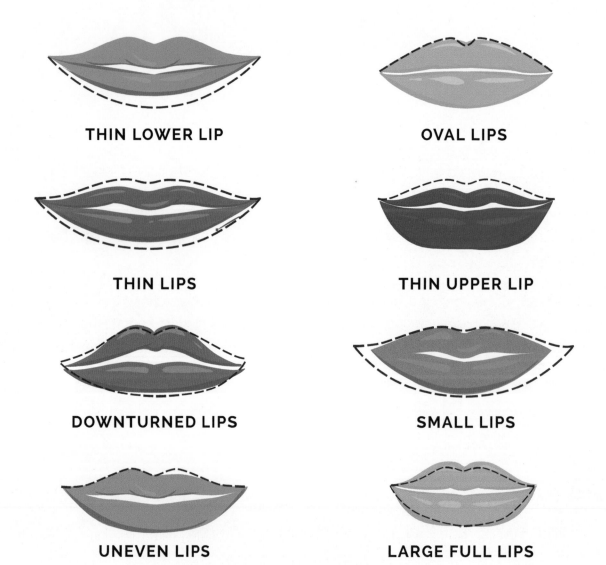

THIN LOWER LIP	**OVAL LIPS**
THIN LIPS	**THIN UPPER LIP**
DOWNTURNED LIPS	**SMALL LIPS**
UNEVEN LIPS	**LARGE FULL LIPS**

"Beauty, to me, is about being comfortable in your own skin. That, or a kick-ass red lipstick."

GWYNETH PALTROW

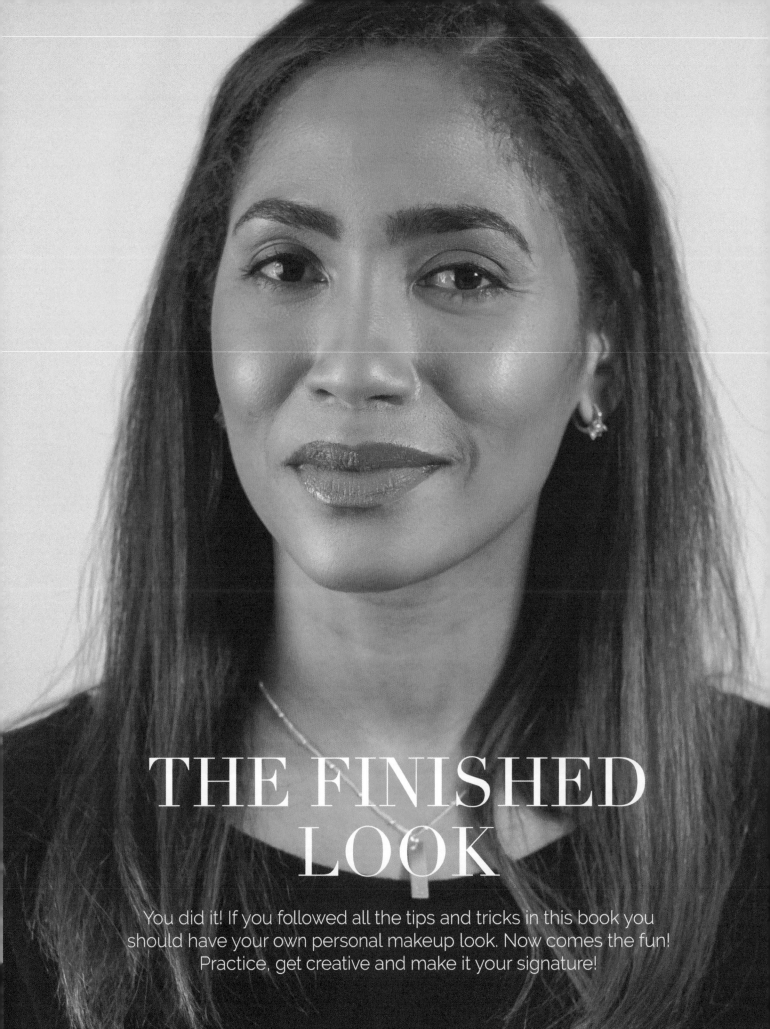

THE FINISHED
LOOK

You did it! If you followed all the tips and tricks in this book you
should have your own personal makeup look. Now comes the fun!
Practice, get creative and make it your signature!

THE END.

Wait, just kidding! **This is really and truly the beginning!**

As you can see, there's no "one size fits all" to makeup. You have learned how to identify your skin type and skin tone, as well as which products may or may not work best for you. We've helped you understand which colors work best on different parts of the face, and given you guidance when it comes to application techniques and tools.

We've covered a lot and yet we've barely scratched the surface! And guess what? Some of what is written in this book may not apply to you. But that's okay!

Hopefully now, you are able to smartly and swiftly navigate through the world of Google searches and YouTube. You know how and where to find information, instead of searching blindly and being overcome by "analysis paralysis."

You know that in addition to becoming intimately familiar with your skin type, undertone, face, eye, eyebrow, and lip shape -- you also have to figure out what types of products work best for your perfect style preferences!

You may have an oval shaped face, cool undertone skin and warm honey eyes that are deep-set and hooded. You could have a heart shaped face that is deep toned with wide-set eyes and full lips. There are so many combinations out there and they're all beautiful in their own way! Like I've said time and time again:

- **Practice makes perfect!**
- **Makeup should be fun!**
- **It's okay to make a mistake, that's what makeup remover is for!**

Once you fall in love with your features, you can decide whether or not you choose to wear makeup. If so, that's great! The techniques you learned will allow you to apply makeup to accentuate your best features (and minimize the ones that make you feel self-conscious). If you decide not to wear makeup—or only wear a little bit... that's fantastic. My goal is to help you see the beauty that is unique to you.

I cannot wait to hear from you and see pictures of your makeup transformations! **With some work and determination, you can be your own makeup artist!**

BOOK CREDITS

I could not have completed this project without the contributions of a team of individuals who offered up their time and talents to make my vision a reality. Thank you to each of you for your support, I couldn't have done it without you!

REFERENCES & CREDITS

COVER & BOOK DESIGN
Kristin Stokes, Moniker Marketing
www.meetmoniker.com
@meetmoniker

IN ORDER OF APPEARANCE

Meredith Davis
Pages 2, 3 (column 1), 25

Anna Dew Photography
Pages 3 (column 2); 15, 21, 27, 46, 62, 90, 94

Greg Kantra
Page 6

FreeStocks.org
Pages 4 (row 2), 26

Kristina Flour
Page 4 (row 3)

Jenelle Botts
Pages 4 (row 4), 29, 32, 34, 37-39, 42, 43, 47, 51, 54, 57, 58, 64, 72 (column 1), 74, 76, 77 (row 2), 82, 88, 99, 102

Jacob Lund
Page 30

Natalie Setareh Personal Collection
Page 36

Leah Knowles
Pages 11, 41, 45, 55, 56, 67, 70, 78, 85, 89, 93

Charisse Kenion
Pages 12, 14

Scott Griessel
Page 48

Peter Hoffmann Photography
Page 61

Wynning Photography
Page 72 (column 2)

Aditya Chhattrala, creativeadi.com
Page 77 (Row 1)

Инна Лаз
Page 80

Sharlotta Ulrikh
Page 84

Cristian Stoian Photography
Page 105

Felicia Buitenwerf
Page 40

Color Theory
Page 34 ©The Flesh Tone Color Wheel™ courtesy of Terri Tomlinson. All rights reserved.

Book
Color Theory for the Make-up Artist: Understanding Color and Light for Beauty and Special Effects, Katie Middleton.

Lipstick Application
Technique learned by KatVonD Master Artist Tara Buenstro at the "Behind TheVeil Bridal Masterclass" at the International Makeup Artist Trade Show in London, 2018.

Makeup History
Face Paint: The Story of Makeup, Lisa Eldridge.

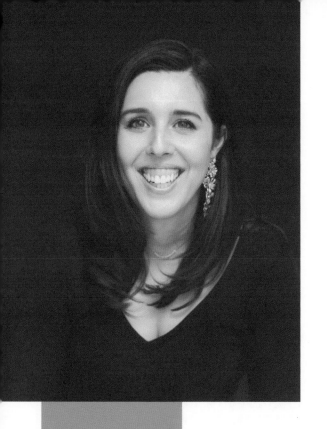

ABOUT NATALIE SETAREH

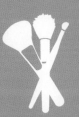

MAKEUP ARTIST

I find such joy in applying makeup on my clients and making them feel amazing through the art of the application. I do not believe in a "one size fits all" makeup application. My passion as a makeup artist is to be mindful of the relationship between the type of makeup I'm applying, as well as the personality of my client.

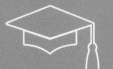

MAKEUP EDUCATOR

I'm tired of the beauty industry convincing people they need to buy everything that comes out. I help people discover the products they really need in my workshops, private lessons, and my exclusive Create Your Signature Look service, designed for non-beauty industry professionals who need to elevate their look.

MAKEUP AFICIONADO

It's true: I eat, sleep, and dream makeup. I have invested so much of my personal time, money, and energy into makeup because it is something that fascinates me. I literally dream of looks for future clients and friends. I can't help but notice makeup trends in my day-to-day life and I love playing with new looks!

Page 105

NS

NATALIE SETAREH

COUTURE MAKEUP ARTIST & BEAUTY COACH

SHARE YOUR BE YOUR OWN MAKEUP ARTIST JOURNEY ONLINE USING:

#BYOMUA

 Stay in touch!
@nataliesetareh

For information on upcoming workshops, unbiased blog posts, makeup tips, tricks and more visit:

www.NatalieSetareh.com

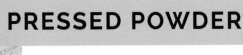

PRESSED POWDER

Don't let the word powder deceive you. Some pressed powders are more full coverage than the fullest coverage foundations in other formulas. Pressed powders are a staple for those of you who hate the feeling of liquid and creams on their face and for shiny foreheads.

- Pressed powders work great for those of you with oily skin.
- They can also be used to "set" foundation for a more full coverage look.
- Apply concealer before you apply your pressed powder foundation!

 Pressed powder is best applied with a tapered natural hair kabuki brush (you can also apply with a velour powder puff). If using a brush, start in the center of the face and apply in small circles (diameter of a cucumber) and lessen the pressure as you move towards your ears.

SERUM FOUNDATION

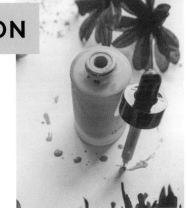

This type of foundation is normally applied directly onto the skin with a dropper or on the fingers and directly onto the face. Serum foundations are generally light to medium coverage. They tend to offer amazing skincare bonuses and do a great job of evening out the skin tone.

  Serum foundation is best applied with the finger tips! Press it in with a sponge to finish.

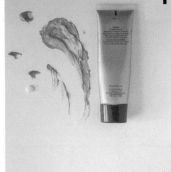

TINTED MOISTURIZER

Tinted moisturizers are such an amazing, versatile day-to-day product. They do a great job of lightly evening out the skin tone, protecting the skin from the sun (most have SPF in them, though you should always wear an actual SPF in addition, okay?), and do not feel (or necessarily look) like you are wearing anything. Apply it over your moisturizer (because #skincare) and mix it with a primer for longevity. **Hint hint!** You can make your own tinted moisturizer by mixing your cream or liquid foundation with your moisturizer.

 Tinted moisturizers can be applied most easily with the fingers and blended with a beauty sponge or buffed in with a brush (optional). Set your tinted moisturizer with a setting powder or powder foundation to intensity the look.

FOUNDATION APPLICATION TIPS

TIP 1: Mixing your foundation with a cream or liquid illuminator (2:1) will help you achieve a dewy, glowing look. You can apply separately or mix your foundation with your favorite moisturizer for a more sheer, natural application.

TIP 2: Remember, you have to add the color and dimension lost through color correction back in, which is covered in the next section.

HOW TO FIND YOUR PERFECT FOUNDATION MATCH...

Visit a store where you can swatch foundations twice; once in summer and once in winter. You'll know your shade when your skin is at its lightest and its darkest, then you can blend the two shades as needed during the bridge seasons. Once you know your shade in one brand, you can more easily shop for dupes!

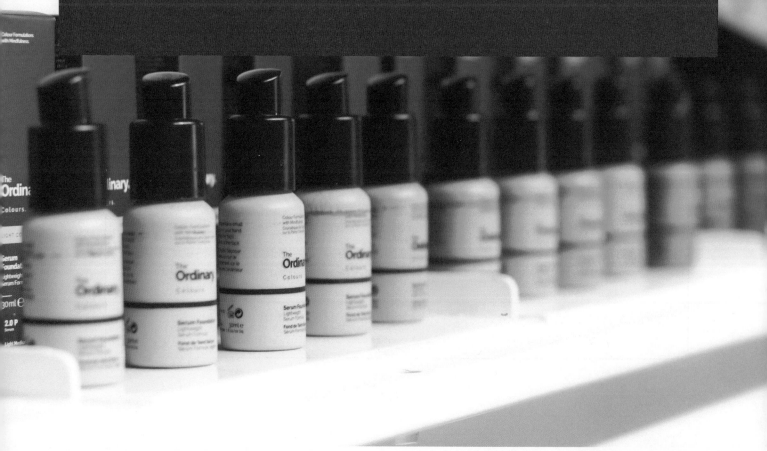